Talking about Sex

Talking about Sex

Sexuality Education for Learners with Disabilities

Elizabeth A. Harkins Monaco,
Thomas C. Gibbon,
and David F. Bateman

ROWMAN & LITTLEFIELD
Lanham • Boulder • New York • London

Published by Rowman & Littlefield
A wholly owned subsidary of The Rowman & Littlefield Publishing Group, Inc.
4501 Forbes Boulevard, Suite 200, Lanham, Maryland 20706
www.rowman.com

Unit A, Whitacre Mews, 26–34 Stannary Street, London SE11 4AB

British Library Cataloguing in Publication Information Available

Library of Congress Cataloging-in-Publication Data

Names: Monaco, Elizabeth A. Harkins, author. | Bateman, David (David F.), author.
Title: *Talking about sex : sexuality education for learners with disabilities* /
    by Elizabeth A. Harkins Monaco, Thomas Gibbons, and David Bateman.
Description: Lanham: Rowman & Littlefield, 2018 | Includes bibliographical references.
Identifiers: LCCN 2017060349 (print) | LCCN 2018002213 (ebook) |
    ISBN 9781475839852 (electronic) | ISBN 9781475839838 (cloth : alk. paper) |
    ISBN 9781475839845 (pbk. : alk. paper)
Subjects: LCSH: Sex instruction for people with mental disabilities. | Sex instruction
    for people with disabilities. | People with disabilities—Sexual behavior.
Classification: LCC HQ54 (ebook) | LCC HQ54 .M656 2018 (print) |
    DDC 306.7087—dc23
LC record available at https://lccn.loc.gov/2017060349

Contents

Preface

In a span of just a few years, adolescents transition dramatically in almost all realms of their lives: they mature physically; their ability to analyze and reason develops; and their social relationships are redefined. Key social and emotional milestones during adolescence are often directly related to the abilities to initiate and maintain intimate relationships (Perkins and Borden 2003), maintain physically maturing bodies, and manage personal sexuality (Murphy and Elias 2006).

Most adolescents with intellectual or developmental disabilities (IDDs) and autism spectrum disorders (ASDs) experience these milestones alongside their neurotypical peers, but they have particular difficulty expressing sexuality in satisfying ways. This population has historically faced issues such as limited intimate relationships, low self-esteem, increased social isolation, deregulated emotional maintenance (Sabornie, Thomas, and Coffman 1989), reduced sexual functioning, and limited sexual health (Blum 1997).

Finding ways to express sexuality is a key part of functional development, and a formal education in sexuality is especially critical for all children but is often neglected for students with IDDs and ASDs (Neufeld et al. 2002). Appropriate sexual knowledge assists not only in achieving personal fulfillment but also in protection from mistreatment, abuse, unplanned pregnancies, or sexually transmitted diseases (STDs) (Murphy and Elias 2006). It also works to help solve problems of loneliness and problems with self-esteem.

Developmentally appropriate sexual knowledge assists not only in achieving personal fulfillment but also in protection from mistreatment, abuse, unplanned pregnancies, or STDs (Murphy and Elias 2006). Additionally, if all stakeholders share the responsibilities for appropriate sexual functioning, students are more apt to adhere to appropriate expectations while maintaining personal safety (Murphy and Elias 2006).

This book will address this but also much more. Issues of physical and cognitive development will be discussed, including appropriate sexual development/urges and brain development, and innate similarities and differences of sexuality that could occur between people with IDs and ASDs, including the complexities of physical disabilities. The authors will also consider special considerations for group homes and recreational facilities and specifically focus on concepts of ethics and models of consent (medical, legal, social, and educational), as well as how to deal with uncertainty. Finally, the text will provide concrete resources for caregivers, parents, and educators who can be directly implemented or modified for use.

Any parent can tell you how hard it is to successfully get an adolescent to delay gratification. For example, think about adolescent requests for the latest phone or video game or their interest in hanging out unsupervised with friends or driving with other young drivers. Parents of children and young adults with disabilities face an even more challenging task. Having a disability does not diminish normal biological human development; adolescents with disabilities develop physically and have sexual desire.

Parents of children with disabilities wrestle with the hopes for their children to have as normal a life as possible while knowing that their children are more likely to be victims of sexual assault. Teaching children with disabilities to negotiate the complex interaction between their developing desires while providing skills for self-protection is particularly problematic if the children have impaired cognitive functioning, emotional instability, impulsivity, or authority aversion (Wissink et al. 2015).

Though this is a topic that many do not want to address, it is clearly of utmost importance. Educating individuals who are vulnerable is a societal interest and one that needs to be taken very seriously. Students with disabilities are at a heightened risk for sexual assault and abuse. Historical trends in our ideology and treatment of people with disabilities as those with fewer rights than other citizens contribute to current vulnerability. Ironically, the normalization movement, with its push for autonomy and self-determination for people with disabilities (PWD), may leave some more vulnerable to not receiving an appropriate education and potentially then suffer from abuse.

REFERENCES

Blum, R. W. (1997). Sexual health contraceptive needs of adolescents with chronic conditions. _Archives of Pediatrics and Adolescent Medicine_, 151: 290–97.

Murphy, N. A., & Elias, E. R. (2006). Sexuality of adolescents with developmental disabilities. _Pediatrics_, 118(1): 398–403.

Neufeld, J. A., Klingbeil, F., Bryen, D. N., & Thomas, A. (2002). Adolescent sexual-
ityand disability. *Physical Medicine and Rehabilitation Clinics of North America*,
13(4): 857–73.

Perkins, D. F., & Borden, L. M. (2003). Positive behaviors, problem behaviors, and
resiliency in adolescence. In R. M. Lerner, M. A. Easterbrooks, & J. Mistry (Eds.),
Handbook of psychology: Volume. 6, Developmental psychology (373–94). New
York: Wiley.

Sabornie, E. J., Thomas, V., & Coffman, R. M. (1989). Assessment of social/affec-
tive measures to discriminate between BD and nonhandicapped early adolescents.
Monograph in Behavior Disorders: *Severe Behavior Disorders in Children and
Youth*, 12: 21–32.

Wissink, I. B., van Vugt, E., Moonen, X., Stams, G. J., & Hendriks, J. (2015).
Sexual abuse involving children with an intellectual disability (ID): A narrative review. *Research in Developmental Disabilities*, 36: 20–35. doi:10.1016/j.
ridd.2014.09.007 PMID:25310832

Acknowledgments

We appreciate the work on the following chapters of these professionals in the field. Their assistance made this book significantly better.

Chapter 3

    Ruth Eyres

Chapter 4

    MaryAnn Shaw

Chapter 5

    Victoria Slocum
    Ruth Eyres

Chapter 6

    Gloria Y. Niles

Chapter 7

    Gloria Y. Niles

Chapter 8

    Rhonda Black

Chapter 10

    Rhonda Black

Chapter 1

Introduction

SUMMARY

In a span of just a few years, adolescents transition dramatically in almost all realms of their lives: they mature physically, their ability to analyze and reason develops, and their social relationships are redefined. Key social and emotional milestones during adolescence are often directly related to the abilities to initiate and maintain intimate relationships (Perkins and Borden 2003), maintain physically maturing bodies, and manage personal sexuality (Murphy and Elias 2006).

A problem is that most adolescents with intellectual or developmental disabilities (IDDs) and autism spectrum disorders (ASDs) have particular difficulty expressing sexuality in satisfying ways, consequently facing issues such as limited intimate relationships, low self-esteem, increased social isolation, deregulated emotional maintenance (Sabornie, Thomas, and Coffman 1989), reduced sexual functioning, and limited sexual health (Blum 1997).

Finding ways to express sexuality is a key part of functional development, and a formal education in sexuality is especially critical for all children but is often neglected for students with IDDs and ASDs (Neufeld et al. 2002). Appropriate sexual knowledge assists not only in achieving personal fulfillment but in protection from mistreatment, abuse, unplanned pregnancies, or sexually transmitted diseases (STDs; Murphy and Elias 2006). It also works to help solve problems of loneliness and self-esteem.

WHO SHOULD BE TAUGHT?

Effective sexuality education for students with IDDs and ASDs must involve the student and stakeholders. Too often sexuality instruction focuses solely

1

on the individual with a disability, but due to the nature of the possible need for long-term supports, others should be included in this education. For many, the education of family and caregivers is just as important and necessary to help the individual with IDD and ASD to develop.

Family Members

Family members are the primary stakeholders in this developmental arena in the earlier ages, but many need assistance when establishing appropriate expectations for their children in relation to cognitive levels, functional abilities, and ages. Many family members have experienced the various stages of development as the individual with IDD or ASD matures, but sexual awareness brings with it other issues, topics, and concerns. Family members are often not prepared to address these concerns and also are unsure about where to go for help (Murphy and Elias 2006).

Much of the instruction for family members has to address preconceived notions and stereotypes. Sexuality instruction should help them understand that while their family member with IDD or ASD may seem to be functioning academically like a first- or second-grade student, significant hormonal changes occur during adolescence. Additionally, adolescents with IDDs or ASDs, and all adolescents, have near-constant exposure to mass and social media including sexually provocative images and associations.

It is not uncommon for family members to talk about "childlike" behaviors that could still include fascination with children's television shows, games, dolls, pets, and even clothing. These activities often preclude thinking about their family member with a developmental disability growing up, getting older, and especially wanting to express himself or herself sexually (Murphy and Elias 2006). Parents may also assume their children are too young or immature to explore appropriate personal sexual preferences or gender norms.

Children with disabilities are capable of—and have the right to—identifying on the gender or sexuality continuum beyond heterosexual or cisgender, but heteronormative assumptions may prevent this. Families need help to realize that their family member will change, that support will need to be provided, and that they will need to address sexuality issues in a way that does not prevent development.

In many respects, the support and acknowledgment of the need for appropriate sexual education for their family member is one of the most important parts of this process. The attitudes, statements, and subsequent actions can have a short- and long-term impact on the ideas and behaviors of the individual with IDD or ASD. Additionally, the opportunities (or nonopportunities) provided by families for spending alone time with a person who may be a sexual partner also will have a long-term impact on the individual with IDD or ASD.

As has been pointed out in many places, the long-term care and support of individuals with IDDs or ASDs often become the responsibility of family members as the parents either become too old or pass away (Brown, McDonnell and Snell 2015). Including the family members helps to ensure a smooth transition and a consistent message. The support of siblings and other family members can be crucial for everyone involved. If home and school share the responsibilities for appropriate sexual functioning, students are more apt to adhere to appropriate expectations while maintaining personal safety (Murphy and Elias 2006).

Just about any parent will tell you how difficult it is to get an adolescent to delay gratification. Think about adolescent requests for the video game, movie, concert tickets, the latest phone, or especially the persistent repeated desire to hang out unsupervised with friends or ride with other young drivers. Parents of children and young adults with disabilities face an even more challenging task. As noted earlier, having a disability does not typically diminish normal biological human development. Just about all adolescents with disabilities develop physically and have sexual desires.

Parents and family members of individuals with disabilities often want their children to have as normal a life as possible, while knowing that their children are more likely to be victims of sexual assault. Teaching children with disabilities to negotiate the increasingly complex interaction between their desires while providing skills for self-protection is particularly problematic if the children have impaired cognitive functioning, emotional instability, impulsivity, or authority aversion.

Balancing a need for development along with the need to help the individual prevent sexual harassment should be an important part of any educational curriculum that is geared toward an individual's needs and ability level. There are programs, agencies, and advocacy groups that provide free information for parents and educators of individuals with disabilities on this topic.

One example, the Florida Developmental Disabilities Council, Inc., provides free educational resources that address topics such as identifying basic body parts, understanding development, and identifying appropriate and inappropriate actions on a level that is easy for students with IDDs to understand (Baxley and Zendell 2005). The Center for Parent Information and Resources (2016) also provides links to information directly related to various disabilities, such as ASDs, deaf-blindness, IDDs, learning disabilities, emotional disturbances, physical disabilities, and traumatic brain injuries. These two resources are just a few of the programs and informational guides that provide education free of charge.

It is important that such information is sought out and delivered to parents and families in a way that will meet their specific needs. The more the parent, caregiver, and family knows about development, appropriate ways to show affection, the right to say no, and then teach ways the individual with a disability can protect themselves from being harmed and/or telling a trusted adult when something inappropriate does occur, the more successful we can be at preventing and stopping sexual assault of individuals with disabilities.

Finally, parents of any adolescent face the multipronged challenge of educating their children about normal biological and human sexual development while warning them about the potential dangers of others. Impulse control in the adolescent brain occurs after brain stem development. The frontal lobes, which also develop later, control impulses and help us to manage behavior; the brain stem sends out messages for the body to act.

Communication between these two parts of the brain is required for carefully considered decision making. Some researchers have suggested that the means of communication between the frontal lobes and brain stem are not completely formed until an individual reaches his or her mid- to late twenties (Marshall and Neuman 2011), further exacerbating the education period related to sexual education.

The Staff

We acknowledge that the first teachers and long-term caregivers and supporters are often family members of the individual with IDD and ASD; however, many individuals require long-term support and care by paid staff. The same statements made about attitudes and perceptions for family members relating to the discussing, instructing, and providing alone time need to be addressed with staff members. Though individuals with IDDs and ASDs may often not require a residential placement and concomitant staff assistance until they are older, the perceptions about childlike behaviors have to be addressed as well.

It is an undisputed problem that we often do not provide sufficient monetary compensation for staff who work with individuals with IDDs and ASDs, and the role they play of in loco parentis is a valuable one; however, we need to realize all of the other demands we often place on them. The other realization that needs to be addressed is the awareness of the frequency of staff turnover, making consistent programs and services often very difficult.

The needs of the individuals with IDDs and ASDs should also be addressed. The important component about this training is ensuring all individuals under their care are treated as individuals. Based on the history of the person with the disability, expectations and comments the individual makes, the expectations and comments made by family members, the location of the services provided, the number of individuals being served, and the interaction with others all provide settings and opportunities that need to be addressed and be individualized.

In addition to all the other responsibilities staff require training about, from billing to confidentiality, to providing appropriate medications to documenting behaviors, staff will need training about issues of sexual education. This training should include terms to use, expectations, and how to respond to certain circumstances. The problem is that training often needs to be provided about the individual needs and expectations for every person with whom they will be working.

The Student

Finally, the needs and desires of the student must be addressed. Like the discussion regarding training the parents and the staff, training about issues of sexuality needs to be individualized to the student. This training needs to address the desires, functioning levels, religious beliefs, and the opportunities that will be presented. There is no one level of education and support appropriate for every individual with IDD or ASD, just like there is no one level of education and support appropriate for individuals who do not have disabilities.

Given the need to individualize the training based about the above descriptors, it is also important to individualize the training based on the comfort level of the student in addressing these issues. For some, the issues are so embarrassing and uncomfortable to talk about that attending or participating in a large-scale class or group on the topic would not be considered an option. Others may be more comfortable and may be more willing to participate in a class and be willing to engage in an open discussion about topics related to sexuality and relationships.

Planning for discussions related to this important topic should include, and will be mentioned repeatedly in later chapters, the need for continuing support to provide information and be available to answer questions as they arise. As will be noted, one-time efforts without follow-up opportunities are inappropriate for topics as important as this. Plan as a part of the instruction for the student, for repeated sessions of information (which may be on the same topic) along with continued availability for questions.

Finally, given all the factors described earlier related to family desires and balanced out with individual desires, education surrounding issues of sexuality may not necessarily occur in schools. For some it may occur in places of worship. Clearly not all individuals participate in regular worship services, so it is inappropriate to assume this is as a sole place of instruction, but for some it is a very important part of their family life.

HISTORY

As unpleasant as it is, it is important to address the history of issues related to sexuality for individuals with disabilities. Some of the attitudes related to sexuality, of which many may be wrong or impractical, may still need to be addressed to help convince family or staff members of the need for education. There is a lot of stigma related to education on issues of sexuality for individuals with developmental disabilities, and many of those stem from historical misconceptions.

The history of sexuality for individuals with disabilities will be covered more extensively in other parts of this book, but they should be a part of any training program that teaches family members and staff about this. The following is a brief background about eugenics, institutionalization, and sexual assault for people with disabilities in order to provide context for the move toward a more comprehensive approach to sexuality education for people with IDDs and ASDs.

Eugenics

Though unpleasant, it is important to discuss the Eugenics Movement. For decades the Eugenics Movement steered much of the discussion related to how we think about individuals with disabilities. This was not just for professionals but pervaded much of the popular media and dramatically altered popular thinking about individuals with disabilities.

The Eugenics Movement and its ideas started to flourish in the late 1800s and were clearly popular until well after World War II and in many respects were still part of the discussion for individuals with disabilities well after that (Allen 2012; Lombardo 2012). The basics of eugenics stemmed from ideas related to how farmers dealt with livestock, where there was a culling of the herd to make the animals stronger by removing the weaker animals, and applying that logic to and belief system to humans (Allen 2012).

Specifically, if reproduction could be controlled so that unfit stock (for farmers) could either be eliminated or at least controlled, then, if applied to humans, problems could be eliminated before they occur; therefore, society would, as a whole, benefit (Allen 2012). The end result would be that we would improve future generations and be able to get rid of undesirable traits (Lombardo 2012).

The observable application of eugenics as applied by farmers with cattle has much more deep-seated roots than that. It was also based on a very narrow and xenophobic interpretation of the Bible (Allen 2012; Lombardo 2012; O'Brien and Bundy 2009). This was extensively used to justify propaganda for years to come afterward.

As the United States went through a series of immigration waves, xenophobia was very present. Along with xenophobia was a prejudice about people with disabilities.

Based on the above, advocates for eugenics increasingly pushed for laws supporting their ideas. In turn, state legislatures started to pass laws based on eugenics, with the first one enacted in 1907 (Lombardo 2012). Increasingly states passed laws sanctioning involuntary sterilization, restricted marriage, and forced institutionalization, with some legislation that supported euthanasia (O'Brien and Bundy 2009).

The main target group for the Eugenics Movement was of those who were "feebleminded," the group we now refer to as individuals with IDDs. Other disability groups were also targeted but to a lesser extent. Those groups included individuals with emotional and behavioral disorders, epilepsy, and sensory impairments (O'Brien and Bundy 2009).

People who were considered feebleminded were the target group because it was believed that all or most cases were due to genetic causes. The intellectual characteristics of individuals who were feebleminded were the ones thought to be undesirable to continue on to other generations. About the same time large institutions to house people with disabilities grew rapidly.

It is sad to point out, that from the 1900s and running through the 1980s, the most common housing placement for people with intellectual disabilities was large state-run institutions. These institutions often resembled hospital campuses and became holding centers. In general, these large institutions did not educate or advance the development of the people with disabilities who lived there. These institutions and their practices were an important outgrowth of the Eugenics Movement.

Families who had children with intellectual disabilities or other disabilities were often told to send their children to the institutions and not encouraged to maintain normal familial connections. There was often no education related to sexuality. There were frequent forced sterilizations, which were easier to carry out in an institutional setting (O'Brien and Bundy 2009).

For our purposes, it is important to point these facts out to highlight how far society has changed (in most places) related to sexual education for individuals with IDDs and ASDs. It is estimated that 65,000 Americans with disabilities were legally sterilized by 1970 (Powell 2014). That number is probably a gross understatement of the true number.

North Carolina recently enacted legislation to compensate the 7,600 residents forced to be sterilized (Thompson 2013). This is the first state to set up this type of compensation system; however, many of the earlier victims are likely deceased. The prevailing thinking was people with disabilities who were institutionalized were not capable of normal human interaction with the opposite sex.

Clearly times have changed, but it is also clear that a lot of work is still left to do.

COMMON SOCIAL ISSUES

Just like the section on eugenics, it is important to point out that problems with sexual assault of individuals with disabilities are all too common. A study released by the U.S. Department of Justice found close to 82,100 cases of rape and/or sexual assault of persons with disabilities were reported each year from 2008 to 2012 (Harrell 2014). The sad part is that the number of reports more than doubled from 2010 to 2011 and the numbers continued to exceed 80,000 reports in 2012 (Harrell 2014).

Another survey, the 2012 National Survey on Abuse of People with Disabilities, found 90 percent of individuals with disabilities who reported some abuse stated abuse was often repeated. Shockingly, 57 percent of these individuals who reported abuse also reported the abuse occurred on more than twenty occasions (Baladerian, Coleman and Stream 2013).

In January 2014, media attention was generated when the White House Council on Women and Girls recognized the increased risk of becoming a victim of sexual assault for individuals with disabilities. This report cites sources indicating individuals with disabilities are three times more likely to experience sexual assault, and women with severe disabilities are four times more likely to be sexually assaulted, when compared to their typically developing peers (White House Council on Women and Girls 2014). Furthermore, Sullivan and Knutson (2000) found children with disabilities were over three times more likely to be the victims of sexual abuse than children without disabilities.

Krohn (2014) recognized this variability in the increased risk across disability groups, age, and gender of individuals with disabilities. Krohn also notes studies have overwhelmingly found women and girls with disabilities show some of the highest percentages of sexual assault victims, stating most females with disabilities experience sexual abuse at some time in their lives. This statement is supported by evidence from the U.S. Department of Justice reports and in a study by Baladerian (1991): 68 percent to 83 percent of women, 39 percent to 83 percent of girls, and 16 percent to 32 percent of boys with developmental disabilities experience sexual assault in their lifetime.

The problem with this data is that it is classically underreported (Wissink et al. 2015). The 2012 National Survey additionally found that 41.6 percent of individuals who took the survey reported sexual abuse, while 41 percent of these victims did not report these incidences to authorities (Baladerian et al. 2013). Krohn also emphasized that cases go unreported, noting that as many as one in thirty survivors with disabilities never report the sexual abuse compared to the one in five survivors without disabilities (Krohn 2014).

Some children who reported sexual assaults said that no action was taken as a result of reporting (Wissink et al. 2015). Also, when incidences were reported to authorities, studies have found low percentages of arrest rates and a high likelihood that no action would be taken as a result of the report. Of all sexual assault and/or rape cases reported in the United States, only 12 percent became investigations between 2005 and 2010 and one study found that cases had been dismissed 75 percent of the time with 80 percent disapproval from the victim (White House Council on Women and Girls 2014).

Getting a good actual number of the risk to people with disabilities is difficult due to the variety of studies on this topic. It is safe to say that children with disabilities are at an increased risk of sexual assault. This is all the more reason for an appropriate and comprehensive education on this topic.

CURRICULUM

The importance of the content of this book cannot be overstated. Individuals with IDDs and ASDs deserve an opportunity to receive not only a free, appropriate public education while they are in school, but they should also receive an education that will help them to understand sexual needs and how to act. As mentioned previously, there needs to be a concerted effort from all parts to help, and that is what this book does.

It is important to highlight the different expectations for the education of students with disabilities in different grades. Sexuality education for students with disabilities is not just a task or responsibility as a part of a secondary education curriculum. Just like other parts of transition instruction, the attitudes and words chosen by elementary teachers also can play a very important role in setting the stage for later more direct and explicit instruction.

As will be presented in this book, we will highlight that sexuality education for students with IDDs and ASDs should be part of a comprehensive curriculum plan and will have four important points guiding all of the chapters as teaching about sexuality is more than just sex education.

1. *Relationships are important.* It is more than just sex. It is about being an important part of someone else's life, which can include living with others.

2. *Respect.* Treating others with respect should be integrated into all training programs, whether relating to sex education or not, but especially when sex is involved—not only respecting others but also respecting oneself and learning to advocate for one's own interests and rights.
3. *Dealing with emotions.* Sex is an emotional response, not just a physical one. We will include discussion items to help individuals with disabilities to address the emotions that come with sex and to help realize this is a very important and often forgotten aspect of the need for training.
4. *Honoring others.* This will build on the ideas of respect and will also make sure that others' opinions and values are treated with dignity and that we do not embarrass others.

While these four points may seem simple, they are actually very important to the overall sexuality education curriculum that needs to be emphasized for individuals not just with IDDs and ASDs but all students. We, however, have the additional responsibility of working to provide an appropriate education for individuals who have historically been not only discriminated against but also legally sterilized and prevented from engaging in sexual activities.

CONCLUSION

Not only is the field of sexual education for individuals with IDDs and ASDs wrestling with the past, it needs help to move forward and pave the way for the future. The various chapters of this book will clarify this.

Specifically, the current best practices in sexual education for individuals with IDDs and ASDs will be highlighted. This will include topics about relationships (of which there are many facets), appropriate sexual developments/urges, public versus private behaviors, safety and personal rights, and curricular adaptations. All of these are very important.

This book will also highlight the changes in adolescent physical and cognitive development, how cognitive development can affect sexual development, family and parent considerations, and information available to parents and families for sexuality education. It will highlight recommendations for teachers and other human services providers, discuss special considerations for group home and recreational facilities, and discuss the similarities (and differences) between IDD and ASD. This text covers consent, issues of self-determination, and dealing with uncertainty, and will conclude with a list of additional resources.

REFERENCES

Allen, A. E. (2012). "Culling the heard": Eugenics and the Conservation Movement in the United States, 1900–1940. *Journal of the History of Biology*, 46: 31–72.

Baladerian, N. (1991). Sexual abuse of people with developmental disabilities. *Sexuality and Disability*, 9(4): 323–335.

Baladerian, N. J., Coleman, T. F., and Stream, J. (2013). *A report on the 2012 national survey on abuse of people with disabilities*. Los Angeles: Spectrum Institute.

Baxley, D. L., and Zendell, A. (2005). *Sexuality education for children and adolescents with developmental disabilities: An instruction manual for caregivers of and individuals with developmental disabilities*. Tallahassee: Florida Developmental Disabilities Council, Inc.

Blum, R. W. (1997). Sexual health contraceptive needs of adolescents with chronic conditions. *Archives of Pediatrics and Adolescent Medicine*, 151: 290–97.

Brown, F. E., McDonnell, J. J., and Snell, M. E. (2015). *Instruction of students with severe disabilities*. Boston: Pearson.

Center for Parent Information and Resources. (2016). *Sexuality education for students with disabilities*. Retrieved November 3, 2017. http://www.parentcenterhub.org/repository/sexed/#materials.

Harrell, E. (2014). *Crimes against persons with disabilities, 2009–1012 statistical tables*. Washington, DC: US Department of Justice.

Krohn, J. (2014). Sexual harassment, sexual assault, and students with special needs: Crafting an effective response for schools. *University of Pennsylvania Journal of Law and Social Change*, 17(1): 2.

Lombardo, P. A. (2012). Return of the Jukes: Eugenic mythologies and Internet evangelism. *American Journal of Legal Medicine*, 33(2): 207–33.

Marshall, R. M., and Neuman, S. (2011). *The middle school mind: Growing pains in early adolescent brains*. Lanham, MD: Rowman and Littlefield.

Murphy, N. A., and Elias, E. R. (2006). Sexuality of adolescents with developmental disabilities. *Pediatrics*, 118(1): 398–403.

Neufeld, J. A., Klingbeil, F., Bryen, D. N., and Thomas, A. (2002). Adolescent sexuality and disability. *Physical Medicine and Rehabilitation Clinics of North America*, 13(4): 857–73.

O'Brien, G. V., and Bundy, M. E. (2009). Reading beyond the "moron": Eugenic control of secondary disability groups. *Journal of Sociology and Social Welfare*, 36(4): 153–71.

Perkins, D. F., and Borden, L. M. (2003). Positive behaviors, problem behaviors, and resiliency in adolescence. In R. M. Lerner, M. A. Easterbrooks, and J. Mistry (Eds.), *Handbook of psychology: Volume. 6, Developmental psychology* (373–94). New York: Wiley.

Powell, R. (2014). Can parents lose custody simply because they are disabled? *GPSolo*, 31(2): 14–17.

Sabornie, E. J., Thomas, V., and Coffman, R. M. (1989). Assessment of social/affective measures to discriminate between BD and nonhandicapped early adolescents.

Monograph in Behavior Disorders: Severe Behavior Disorders in Children and Youth, 12: 21–32.

Sullivan, P.M., and Knutson, J.F. (2000). Maltreatment and disabilities: A population-based epidemiological study. *Child Abuse & Neglect*, 24(10): 1257–1273.

Thompson, J. (2013). A historical earmark, *Nation*, 297: 5.

White House Council on Women and Girls (2014). *Rape and sexual assault: A renewed call to action.* Washington, DC: Author.

Wissink, I. B., van Vugt, E., Moonen, X., Stams, G. J., and Hendriks, J. (2015). Sexual abuse involving children with an intellectual disability (ID): A narrative review. *Research in Developmental Disabilities*, 36: 20–35. DOI:10.1016/j.ridd.2014.09.007 PMID:25310832.

Chapter 2

We're in This Together: Who Are the Educators?

The World Health Organization (WHO) indicates that

> sexual health is a state of physical, emotional, mental and social well being in relation to sexuality; it is not merely the absence of disease, dysfunction or infirmity. Sexual health requires a positive and respectful approach to sexuality and sexual relationships, as well as the possibility of having pleasurable and safe sexual experiences, free of coercion, discrimination and violence.

Parents and educators are more likely to identify with the following: *My son can't do basic math! How is he going to pick out a girlfriend or boyfriend?* Or *How can my daughter choose a partner when she can't choose the right shoes to wear?* Or *Picking a good partner is difficult for everyone. Even I've been divorced.*

SUMMARY

Understanding the responsibilities and consequences of sexuality ultimately defines one's abilities to make safe and healthy decisions as adults. When accurate and developmentally appropriate information is presented, people become more capable of protecting their health and exhibiting less risky behavior by developing skills that manage conflict, improve basic communication, and generalize strategies (FoSE 2017). This is especially more complicated for students with intellectual or developmental disabilities (IDDs) and autism spectrum disorders (ASDs).

Exploring different belief systems, promoting dialogues about sexual values—religious, cultural, and social considerations—and providing necessary skills training in a variety of settings are best done collaboratively when educators and families work together to shape their roles. Developing mutually agreed-upon values promotes interactive dialogues, skill development, and diverse opportunities for practice. A collaborative approach empowers students to gain control over this intimate area of development through self-validation, personal expression, and meaningful understanding of personal sexuality (MacRae 2013).

If all members of the education team work together to identify expertise in skill development alongside content that is comfortable and accessible, they can best modify and adapt the available curriculum and resources.

The following can guide practitioner collaboration and readers will be able to provide:

- ways to routinely discuss sexuality as skills, behaviors, or activities of daily living (ADLs).
- opportunities for parents/caregivers and educators to gain the knowledge and skills (accessible and convenient).
- parents/caregivers and their children with opportunities to practice.
- approaches that promote family and educator involvement.
- opportunities to share information and value systems.

(SIECUS, 2002)

PARENTS AS EDUCATORS

All children are exposed to messages about modesty, nudity, and privacy; gender-specific proper conduct; the acknowledgment and discussion of physical differences between men and women; and the use and response of sexual language; many of these messages are intrinsically relayed by parents and caregivers and shape children's awareness of sexuality at young ages. They also impact children's personal development of value systems, appropriate behaviors, and the understanding of explicit and implicit messages and actions.

Despite parents' critical importance in shaping this development, it is natural for them to feel uncomfortable. It is vital then that they are equipped to strategically choose their levels of involvement in their children's sexuality, especially considering adults with IDDs and ASDs often require increased parental supervision beyond adolescence. "There is often a need for parents . . . to be involved in facilitating with transportation and arrangements" (Walker-Hirsh 2007, 87).

This increased level of involvement has consequences for the children however, as limited opportunities for privacy, safe experimentation, access to appropriate peers, and innate challenges with social pragmatics often result in poor or unsafe decision making. Common mistakes include choosing inappropriate locations or times for sexual activity or participation in activities for which they are not emotionally prepared. "Ultimately, caring parents and their children [need to] make the effort required to come to terms with the extent and the ways in which sexuality can be incorporated successfully into their lives" (Walker-Hirsh 2007, 92).

Overall while most families believe sexual education is important for students with IDDs and ASDs, many do not support the implementation of instruction (Walker-Hirsh 2007). Research suggests parents fear that if instruction is provided, students will become confused or act inappropriately; that their children are not in need of a formal sexuality education; or that content is concerned only with male and female anatomy or the act of intercourse.

While adolescence is an incredibly significant time period for all children, we cannot underestimate its importance for parents. "The discrepancy between the hopes and plans that parents have for their children before a diagnosis of disability and the adaptations that will be required as a result of that diagnosis is repeated and takes on a different face at each new stage of maturity. The pain of parents' awareness of their child's limitations and the implications of those limitations for the parents is repeated at each new stage of growth and development" (Walker-Hirsh 2007, 79).

Any noticeable anxiety or discomfort will encourage avoidance of certain topics, which in time only amplifies feelings of anxiety in their children. *The sooner parents are ready for implementing appropriate sexuality training in their child's lives, the better.* "Language for discussion, when it has not already been established during childhood, is more difficult to introduce when the child is more sexually aware and when silences has already been the established level of communication" (Walker-Hirsh 2007, 77). When parents are able to set aside any personal fears, they are better able to understand that academic or intellectual progress is not necessarily indicative of developmental maturity.

Subculture Norms

Access to helpful strategies and shared successful practices help determine the degree to which one should appropriately intervene with their children's sexual development (Walker-Hirsh 2007). "The solidarity and permanence of a strong support system should be assured before an adult with [IDD or ASD] and his or her parents make decision[s]" (Walker-Hirsh 2007, 84). Strong cultural networking systems can naturally address these sometimes-awkward topics.

Subcultures, the values and norms of minority subgroups, create communities of people who collectively focus on the resolve of personal societal problems by developing value systems that are reinforced by mutually shared characteristics. In fact, when groups strongly identify, members become increasingly dependent on each other for social contact and validation of their beliefs and ways of life.

At the core then, parents of children with IDDs and ASDs belong to a subculture of other parents of children with IDDs and ASDs. This arena provides parents opportunities to discuss personal value systems as related to their children's sexual health. The influence of this subculture on sexuality education arguably then is unparalleled (Walker-Hirsh 2007).

Parent Dos and Don'ts

The first step for families can be as simple as identifying personal belief systems:

1. Define personal belief systems.
2. Identify comfortable and uncomfortable topics.
3. Identify alternative belief systems.
4. Accept that all children, *regardless of cognitive abilities*, deserve opportunities to determine personal sexuality philosophies, belief systems, and rules for personal sexuality.
5. Seek out factual information about sexuality prior to having any discussions.
6. Encourage children to record any personal interests or questions to address later.

Table 2.1 describes strategies that focus on building a skills-based foundation for mature topics of discussion, rather than on specific topics of sexuality. Table 2.2 describes recommendations for family standards and expectations about sexuality. Table 2.3 provides recommendations for school and family responsibilities regarding sexuality education.

Table 2.1   Recommendations for Family Discussions about Sexuality

Dos *with your children*	**Don'ts** *with your children*
• Discuss sexuality openly—start early!	• React in anger
• Research factual answers	• React in fear
• Be sensitive to child's needs	• Refuse to discuss topics of interest
• Ask questions like, "Why are you asking? Where did you hear that? Were you talking about this with anyone else?	• Shame the child or laugh at your child's questions or comments
	• Create an authoritative environment
• Answer with facts	• Assume your child is not aware of topics of sexuality
• Use reassurance	
• Bring up topics of concern for discussion, even if your child is unaware of topics	• Ignore elements of peer or media influences on your child's knowledge of sexuality

(Walker-Hirsh, 2007)

Table 2.2　Family Standards and Expectations about Sexuality

Do have high standards for . . .	*By expecting them to . . .*
Social behavior	– act appropriately according to age (interests, behavior, decorum, etc.) – identify a plan to react and problem-solve in age-appropriate ways – compromise with others on a variety of topics and/or activities
Self-advocacy	– ask for what they want or need – articulate how they feel – ask questions about personal sexuality – ask questions about sexuality concepts
Self-determination	– practice making decisions and choices on a multitude of personal topics – make decisions and choices that properly address personal maturity and sexuality – problem-solve through challenging moments
Self-reflection	– think about his/her personal beliefs – ask questions about family belief systems – determine personal sexuality beliefs

Table 2.3　School and Family Responsibilities Regarding Sexuality Education

Dos *with the school*	**Don'ts** *with the school*
• Discuss sexuality openly • Ask counselor or special educator for social and behavioral evaluation • Identify home responsibilities • Identify school responsibilities • Identify "deal breaker" topics and determine appropriate personnel to address them • Seek out informal and formal resources (school- or community-based) • Seek out curriculum and resources	• React in anger • React in fear • Refuse to discuss topics of interest • Shame the child or laugh at the child's questions or comments • Refuse to collaborate • Ignore or disregard alternative sexuality curriculum that does not align with personal values • Refuse to generalize school skills at home

Remember, There Is Not One Correct Answer!

A cohesive, collaborative plan helps parents better equip themselves in assisting their children. A natural first step to this process is to initiate a conversation with the education team:

EDUCATOR RESPONSIBILITIES

Educators may struggle expediting comprehensive sexuality training. Similarly to parents, they may feel anxious or overwhelmed, or not understand where to start, what to teach, or when to address certain concepts. A teacher may or may not be aware of his or her own biases about sexuality, or not have much knowledge about the biological, emotional, or legal aspects of sexuality. In addition, many do not have clear-cut guidelines for classroom discussion of sensitive or ethical subjects.

Comprehensive approaches to sexuality education prevent sexual violence and premature pregnancy through teaching effective ways to understand and identify healthy and unhealthy relationship patterns and personal needs. The impact of this is critical. Teenagers who receive comprehensive sexuality education are 50 percent less likely to experience pregnancy than those who received abstinence-only programs. "Most Western European countries now have mandatory, comprehensive sexuality education, and consequently have lowered their adolescent pregnancy rates to fewer than 40 per 1,000" (Davies and Dubie 2012, 1).

Unfortunately however, "the United States, Russia, Bulgaria, Belarus, and Romania (all of which restrict or delay sexuality education) have rates of more than 70 per 1,000" (Davies and Dubie 2012, 1). While there is a national dialogue in the United States about appropriate sexuality education, it is required in only twenty-two states and Washington, DC. Only nineteen of those states require medical, factual, or technically accurate curriculum; some states ban discussions about contraceptives or abortion or mandate abstinence and heterosexuality-focused instruction (Blad 2014). Arguably, people with IDDs and ASDs are likely more adversely affected by abstinence-only approaches and the traditional way sexuality education has been taught in the school systems.

If educators are uncomfortable or don't feel capable of teaching sexuality education, they are sending messages almost as strong as giving the wrong information. "This fact is perhaps the single most important consideration in understanding and successfully implementing sexuality education for students with [IDD and ASD]" (Walker-Hirsh 2007, 5). Defining appropriate and comfortable involvement is critical. Remember, the teacher's tone and chosen content could be the only accurate and nonjudgmental information students receive!

School Policies

Recent data shows many schools do not prepare students for puberty, and teaching sexuality is less common than what teachers feel necessary. In addition, there is a lack of fiscal support. Since 1996, federal funding has distributed over a billion dollars to programs promoting abstinence, while comprehensive sexuality programs do not have access to equal funding.

Furthermore, sexuality education teachers report feeling unsupported by the community, parents, or administrators, and express a need for more professional training (Landry, Singh, and Darroch 2000).

Permissions

The Future of Sex Education (FoSE) Initiative, a partnership between Advocates for Youth, Answer, and the Sexuality Information and Education Council of the United States (SIECUS), proposed new sexuality standards in June 2014, to provide teachers with resources to navigate sexuality in the classroom. FoSE offers specific examples addressing common difficulties in sexuality education, such as prevention of sexually transmitted infections (STIs) in places where state laws emphasize abstinence. FoSE advises how to consult not only state law and formal school policies but also how to directly access administrative support to determine how to teach more comprehensively while stressing elements of the law (Blad 2014). (FoSE standards are available in chapter 11).

Seeking guidelines for behavioral issues as related to sexuality can help teachers navigate difficulties with public masturbatory behavior, self-stimulating behavior, inappropriate touching of others, or intimate behavior. Remember, by focusing more on elements of "social inclusion, sexual safety, and life enjoyment," opportunities to incorporate instruction beyond abstinence can increase (Walker-Hirsh 2007, 5). The following checklist outlines concrete information that teachers can easily seek out:

- Definition of sexuality
- Legal implications
- Behavioral concerns
  - inappropriate self-touch
  - public and private places
  - inappropriate and appropriate clothing
  - allowable sexual expression
- Basic hygiene
  - menstruation
  - toileting skills
- Sexual orientation
- Gender identification
- Sexual mistreatment or abuse
- STIs and other sexually transmitted diseases
  - HIV/AIDS
  - Zika

Special Education Law

In 1975, Congress passed Public Law 94–142 (Education of All Handicapped Children Act), which guaranteed a free, appropriate public education (FAPE) to children with disabilities on a national scale. Amendments to the law and eventual changes led to the Individuals with Disabilities Education Act (IDEA) in 2004, No Child Left Behind (NCLB) in 2002, and Every Student Succeeds Act (ESSA) in 2015. These laws emphasize that students with disabilities have the same educational opportunities to the maximum extent possible as typically developing peers, but they do not specify specific curricula addressing sexuality (Lang, Erikson and Jones 2001).

If the school does not believe sexuality curriculum is part of its obligation under federal law, perhaps the sections of special education law outlining transition planning as the process for achieving productive and meaningful lives can be referenced. A fully integrated livelihood in adulthood goes beyond traditional academics, and the law emphasizes the importance of social and emotional fulfillment (CFR 34 §300.305). Going out into the world with sexual ignorance or vulnerability to predation is not consistent with the requirements of a comprehensive transition process.

The Special Education Team

Given the comprehensive nature of sexuality, integrating skill development alongside opportunities for appropriate content and social sexual expression is critical. When students have opportunities to express ideas, make decisions, and solve problems across a number of settings utilizing a combination of skills, they are better able to contribute to personal psychosocial development, uphold a basic sense of well-being, and increase socialization. Students with IDDs and ASDs can better access curriculum that is augmented individually by learning from specialists' expertise in matching specialized skills to the specialized needs of the students.

Special educators not only are in the unique position of coordinating the special education team but are also cognizant of their student's unique needs and abilities and are well positioned to support decisions being made about when, how much, and specific content of the sexuality information a young person should receive. Special educators by trade are able to actively involve more than just content and include skills needed to utilize knowledge in a meaningful way.

They can also determine appropriate skills that are better addressed by service providers (e.g., specialized teachers, speech therapists, occupational therapists, physical therapists, paraprofessionals, social workers), who are essential in creating individualized education plans encompassing specific areas of skill development.

Occupational therapists, for example, can determine appropriate ADLs within sexuality, such as basic hygiene, the physical capabilities of being sexually satisfied, or the development of leisure interests; speech pathologists could focus on the development of empathy, sensitivity, and communication within sexuality, relationships, and advocacy; and school counselors, psychologists, or social workers could provide therapeutic interventions to help students achieve goals of sexual expression and satisfaction, or the expression of fears, concerns, or needs.

General Educators

Sexuality education is often taught by general health or physical education teachers who have had little or no training on human sexuality, legal or ethical issues, classroom-management concerns, or strategies to best educate students with IDDs or ADDs. A 2010 study found only 61 percent of colleges and universities require sexuality education courses for preservice health educators, and nearly a third of sexuality education teachers reported no preservice or in-service training (Blad 2014). Among the institutions that do require sexuality coursework, many only require a general survey course focusing only on content and not on issues related to teaching it (Blad 2014).

Despite limited training, health and physical education providers are considered the in-service experts in research-based resources and supports, authentic content, and skill-development strategies. At the minimum, health and physical education teachers have access to school resources and curricula directly aligning with the school district's sexuality policies, and can maximize opportunities for collaboration within the regular education classroom.

HOW CAN YOU STAY CURRENT ON THIS TOPIC?

Five cohesive steps can begin the process of developing a comprehensive sexuality education plan. The first step is to *contact the parents* (example letters are provided in chapter 11). Then, *conduct a needs assessment*, seeking specific skills-based information, while working to *gather support* and *research solutions* among the stakeholders. Don't forget to include *individual student needs alongside school policies*. Then, *gather available resources*, *develop a plan,* and *create or modify a curriculum* (Planned Parenthood 2017). Table 2.4 provides details about potential next steps in developing sexuality education.

Additional resources for writing curriculum are discussed in chapter 4. Specific resources are provided in chapter 11.

Table 2.4 Steps to Develop a Sexuality Education Plan

Conduct a Needs Assessment	Assess personal attitudes, values, and belief systems. Create a safe learning environment. Identify gaps and needs in the students' knowledge. Identify gaps and needs in the students' skills. Develop and practice a protocol for answering difficult questions. Develop and implement an evaluation plan. Develop and implement a plan to get feedback from all stakeholders.
Gather Support	Identify the stakeholders: • parents/caregivers • education team (special educators, regular educations, specialists/ service providers, paraprofessionals) • administrators • community leaders • health care professionals • students Involve stakeholders early in the process: • Identify culturally appropriate content. • Harvest support among stakeholders. Offer stakeholders opportunities to determine and evaluate content. Train stakeholders to communicate with the children about sexuality issues.
Research Solutions	Research what is already being done on this topic by the home, school, organization, or community. Partner with other experienced professionals. Research and select an established, evaluated sexuality education curriculum or develop your own.
Gather Available Resources	Review various teaching methodologies. Define necessary content. Incorporate differentiated and multimodal approaches into each lesson plan. Seek out appropriate professional development opportunities.
Develop a Plan and Create or Modify a Curriculum	Use state department of education, school board policies, and SIECUS. Balance the content of your lessons with the need to *convey information* and *develop skills*. Carve out adequate time to implement lessons. Develop homework assignments and activities that provide opportunities for families to practice skills, share values, and reinforce facts. Empower students to communicate appropriately about sexuality.

(SIECUS, 2002).

CONCLUSION

Despite the widely recognized importance of sexual health, sexuality education remains sensitive and sometimes controversial, especially for students with IDDs and ASDs. The content of sexuality education, the identification of primary stakeholders in sexuality education, and the innate skill differences of students with IDDs and ASDs further complicate this discussion. Sexual health education programs must be designed to meet individual needs and is not the exclusive domain of parents or educators; rather, collaboration between home and school best provides adolescents with the tools they need to improve their sexual health in adulthood.

Sexuality, the exploration of ourselves, specifically with our physical bodies, our emotions, our self-worth and image, and our interrelations with others, is one of the most basic human instincts and a natural part of human development, but incredibly complicated. Many other factors impact personal sexual growth and development including where, when, and how one is raised, by whom, personal value systems, and access to a sexuality curriculum (WHO 2010). These factors, when combined with developmental aspects beyond biology (social, emotional, educational, and intellectual processing), are often difficult for children—especially those with disabilities—to navigate independently.

REFERENCES

Blad, E. (2014). New teacher-preparation standards target sex education. *Education Week*, 33(30): 14.

Davies, C., and Dubie, M. (2012). *Intimate relationships and sexual health: A curriculum for teaching adolescents/adults with high-functioning autism spectrum disorders and other social challenges.* Lenexa, KS: AAPC Publishing.

Future of Sex Education (FoSE). (2017). *Youth health and rights in sex education.* Retrieved January 9, 2017, from http://www.futureofsexed.org/youthhealthrights. html on January 9, 2017.

Individuals with Disabilities Education Act. (1997). CFR 34 §300.305.

Landry, D. J., Singh, S., and Darroch, J. E. (2000). Sexuality education in fifth and sixth grades in U.S. public schools, 1999. *Family Planning Perspectives*, 32(5): 21.

Lang, D., Erikson, J., and Jones, K. (2001). Kansas works to meet the needs of special education students. *SIECUS Report*, 29(3): 26.

MacRae, Nancy (2013). Sexuality and the role of occupational therapy. *American Journal of Occupational Therapy*, 62: 625–83. DOI:10.5014/ajot.62.6.625.

Planned Parenthood. (2017). Fact Sheets and Reports. https://www.plannedparenthood.org/about-us/newsroom/fact-sheets-reports.

SIECUS. (2002). Fact Sheets. Retrieved November 3, 2017. http://siecus.org/index.cfm?fuseaction=Page.ViewPage&pageId=621.

Walker-Hirsh, L. (2007). *The facts of life . . . and more: Sexuality and intimacy for people with intellectual disabilities*. Baltimore, MD: Paul H. Brooks Publishing.

World Health Organization. (2010). Sexual Health (Fact Sheet Health Topics). http://www.who.int/topics/sexual_health/en/.

Chapter 3

The Birds and the Bees:
Specific Skills and
Teaching Strategies

The importance of sexuality education for people with IDD and ASD can-
not be overemphasized for not only safety of individuals, but also quality
of life—isn't it human nature to desire full and satisfying adulthood?

—Leslie Walker-Hirsch, *The Facts of Life . . . and More*

SUMMARY

Skills that increase responsible, independent decision making about personal safety are crucial in sexuality. Skill basics not only support puberty and development, but they are also essential in promoting the right to decide *what behaviors to engage in* and how to *say no to unwanted sexual activity*. Regardless of cognitive capabilities, irresponsible sexual activities and choices have serious consequences, both physical and emotional. Sexual relationships are often idiosyncratic and abstract, therefore requiring a higher level of abstract thinking in order to sufficiently generalize information.

In order for relationships to be accessible and meaningful, we must help individuals access "numerous opportunities to develop specific language, role-playing opportunities as rehearsal, numerous chances to practice . . . in a supportive environment, and support in planning the activity and logistics" (Walker-Hirsch 2007, 15). This is best addressed through the development of self-determination, social pragmatics, and emotional maintenance, and is especially critical for individuals with IDDs and ASDs.

After reading this chapter, readers will be able to identify:

- basic skills and skill development for self-determination, social pragmatics, and emotional maintenance;

- teaching strategies to best embed these skills in the classroom;
- adaptive tools; and
- the importance of generalization.

SELF-DETERMINATION

The Convention on the Rights of Persons with Disabilities was updated to prohibit compulsory sterilization of individuals with disabilities and guarantee the right to adopt children (United Nations 2006). A focus on including family rights in the Convention influenced familial and public perception toward seeing persons with disabilities as fully human, with rights to make their own decisions regarding sexual reproduction and/or creating a family through adoption. A basic understanding that persons with disabilities are fully human is crucial in offering opportunities to acquire self-determination skills.

Multiple studies have indicated students with higher levels of self-determination are more likely to fare better in life, including independent living, self-advocacy, and decision making (Taylor, Richards, and Brady 2005; Wehmeyer and Palmer 2003). Including self-determination as a component of comprehensive sexuality education is helpful because having greater independence and control of one's life through decision making (Travers et al. 2014) is a crucial part of learning the skills necessary to make personal sexual decisions.

Self-determination includes many important skills all persons encounter on a daily basis: choice making, problem solving, setting goals, and evaluating options (National Parent Center on Transition and Employment 2016). For most individuals, opportunities readily exist to practice these skills (e.g., selecting clothing, seasoning food, setting up social events or meetings with friends, deciding when/where to eat, deciding on jobs/volunteer work, navigating what to do when the A/C unit does not work).

Unfortunately, many young people with IDDs and ASDs have limited opportunities to practice such skills. A need exists for opportunities to be offered that include choice making, positive self-perceptions, and making decisions about life through choice-making, goal setting, self-monitoring, and self-advocacy (Taylor et al. 2005; Travers et al. 2014).

Self-determination theory (figure 3.1) explains that competence, autonomy, and relatedness are the three basic psychological needs of all humans (Ryan and Deci 2000). Similarly, the field of special education outlines self-determination as the learning and acquiring autonomy, self-regulation, and self-realization (Wehmeyer and Fields 2007), which ultimately helps individuals exercise choice and control in their everyday lives. Providing

Self-Determination Theory

Autonomy
need to control
the course of their
life

Competence
need to be
effective in
dealing with
environment

Relatedness
need to have close,
affective
realtionships with
others

3
basic
human
needs

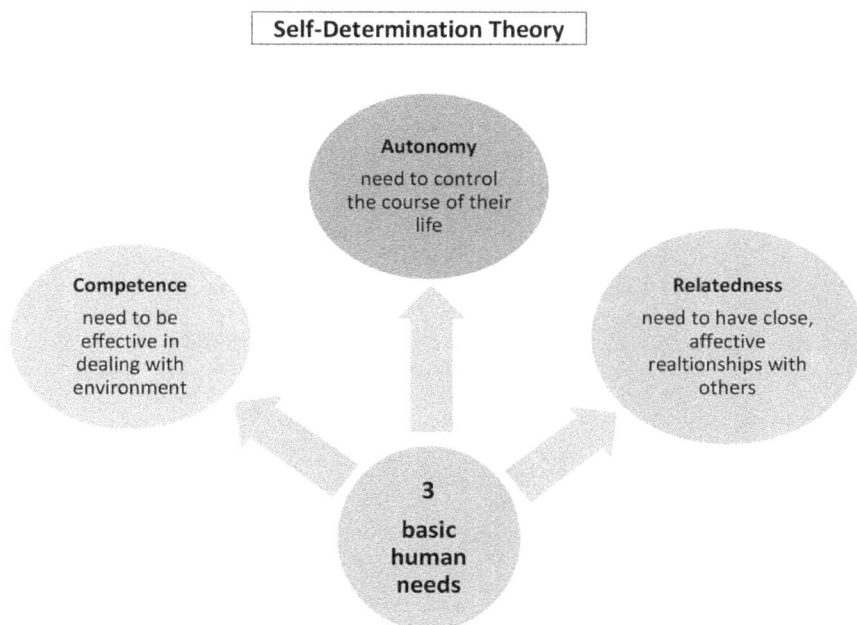

Figure 3.1   Self-Determination Theory

instruction-teaching skills in self-determination to students with IDDs and ASDs establishes a foundation on which to teach sexuality education concepts.

Teaching Self-Determination

Table 3.1 presents ideas about how to incorporate skills important for teaching self-determination to persons with IDD and ASD.

Including sexuality education concepts into self-determination instruction often presents barriers for families and educators. Personal beliefs, stereotypes, and fear often prevent access to sexuality education for individuals with developmental disabilities (Wilkenfeld and Ballan 2011). Table 3.2 offers sexuality education topics related to self-determination and strategies/ materials to use for instruction.

SOCIAL PRAGMATIC SKILLS

Many individuals with IDDs and ASDs are at higher risks to confront social situations with problematic behaviors, such as disruption, aggressiveness, isolation, or anxiety, and ultimately experience the loss of reciprocal

Table 3.1 Recommendations to Help Students Build Self-Determination Skills

In order to help students . . .	*Teach this:*
Make choices	• Choice within an activity • Choice between two or more activities • Deciding when to do an activity • Selecting the individual with whom to participate in an activity • Selecting where to do an activity • Refusing to do an activity • Choosing to terminate an activity at a self-selected time (Brown, Appel, Corsi, and Wenig 1993)
Make decisions	• Deciding if there is a problem and how you feel • Thinking about all the choices you have • Knowing what will happen with each choice and deciding if the choice meets your goals • Deciding which choice is best for you and making a decision (Wehmeyer 2007, 48)
Problem-solve	• Identify problem • Create a mental representation • Work through the problem • Solve and evaluate • Reflect (do2learn.com 2017)
Set goals	• Student identifies something they wish to work toward • Student develops a plan to reach that particular objective • Ensure objectives are challenging, yet feasible and aligned to their likes and dislikes (Cabeza et al. 2013)
Self-monitor	• Come to consensus with the student on the definition of the target behavior • Develop a simple self-monitoring form • Set a goal for (and with) the student • Provide consistent reinforcement for meeting the goal or correctly monitoring the behavior (Bell, Magill, Carter, and Lane 2013)

relationships in both school and the community (Gilliam 2005). They typically have difficulties understanding that other perspectives are different from their own or are not able to read facial expressions or body language. People with IDDs and ASDs may misinterpret the use and meaning of vocal inflections or the use of personal space (Gallagher 1991), leading to inaccurate conclusions or inappropriate reactions.

If individuals do not understand questions or comments, their responses may seem silly or unintelligent; others may overreact with angry words or actions, or not react at all when a response is required or expected, causing confusion or frustration with their conversation partners (Gallagher 1991).

Adolescents depend on intimate relationships with others to help regulate personal social and emotional development; adolescents with IDDs and

Table 3.2   Recommendations to Help Students Build Self-awareness, Safety Skills, Personal Rights, and Self-advocacy

In order to help students learn . . .	*Teach this:*	*Use this:*
Self-awareness	• Personal care/hygiene • Autonomy • Relationships (friendship, dating, marriage) • Healthy choices (Eyres, Williamson, Hunter, and Casey 2016)	• Hygiene kits • Preference assessments • Pictures of family, friends, teachers, etc. • Visual sequences of personal care steps
Safety and personal rights	• Public vs. private • How to say no • Consent (The Healthy Bodies Toolkit 2013)	• Public behavior pictures • Private behavior pictures • Role-play
Self-advocacy	• Personal space • Communicating preferences, desires, and opinions • Interpersonal communication skills (Cabeza et al. 2013)	• Hula hoop to visualize personal space • Participation in IEP conferences

ASDs aren't any different. They too struggle with the adjustment to new social demands of adolescence and are at higher risk of social isolation (Perkins and Borden 2003). Different types of communication are necessary in order to lead fulfilling lives in which one is able to express feelings of love and friendship appropriately. Friendships and romantic relationships—including the intricacies of dating, love, and marriage—are possible only when the complexities of social skills are developed.

Expressive and Receptive Language

Expressive language is a broad term describing how people communicate their personal wants and needs. It encompasses verbal and nonverbal communication skills and the use of language. Expressive language skills include facial expressions, gestures, intentionality, vocabulary, semantics (word/sentence meaning), linguistics, and syntax (grammar rules).

Receptive language includes the ability to comprehend language, including attention, listening, and processing to gain information. Areas of receptive language skills include receptive vocabulary, following directions, and understanding elements of language (answering questions).

Nonverbal communication consists of up to 80 percent of overall communication and includes facial expressions, gestures, and body language. These elements, as well as facilitating awareness and change in interactions based on general social rules and norms, make up *social pragmatic skills* and are absolutely vital when developing and maintaining friendships (ASHA 2017).

The importance of developing social skills cannot be overstated; the combination of expressive and receptive language, nonverbal communication, and an understanding of social norms are absolutely critical when establishing healthy sexual behaviors. This is especially challenging for people with ASDs and IDDs, who are not only excluded from social participation but also experience sexual exclusion.

Teaching Social Skills

Only when social pragmatic skills are mastered can individuals more easily develop and engage in verbal and nonverbal communication, and determine appropriate reactions to social situations. The intricate combination of social pragmatic skills is challenging for students with IDDs and ASDs, especially when considering sexual relationships—whether with oneself or others.

Parents/caregivers and teachers can support social pragmatics by consulting with the student's speech and language pathologist, especially to identify teaching strategies, resources, and ideas for generalization. Then, the next step is to determine the strategies the classroom teacher and caregivers/parents are capable of—such as *direct teaching, opportunities for generalization* alongside *visuals, hands-on manipulatives*, and a variety of *low or high technological tools*. Table 3.3 can help get you started:

Table 3.3   Recommendations to Help Students Build Social Pragmatic Skills

In order to help students . . .	*Teach this:*	*Use this:*
Express wants, needs, thoughts, and ideas	• Opportunities to speak and time to rehearse before speaking • Vocabulary lists to help with word-finding difficulties. Use appropriate and consistent vocabulary • Small group work to give children confidence to express themselves • Word play • Storytelling • Discussing what they have seen or done with an adult or more verbally able peer	• Visual clues to help order ideas effectively • Visual scripts • Rhymes • Picture boards • Magnetic words or letters • Specific writing or dictation tools • Assistive technology computer programs/electronic devices

In order to help students . . .	Teach this:	Use this:
Argue a point of view	• Revise links and associations between ideas and vocabulary—categories and function; context/similarity/ association	• Color-coding different groups of words/sets of pictures • Specific writing or dictation tools • Assistive technology computer programs/electronic devices
Develop use of language in writing	• Giving correct models of language structures • Repetition and reinforcement of correct language structures	• Picture boards • Magnetic words or letters • Assistive technology computer programs/electronic devices
Understand verbal language from others	• Restrict your language to short unambiguous language • Appropriate questioning to give children the opportunities to reply	• Visual clues • Visual scripts • Rhymes • Picture boards
Understand gestures and facial expressions to communicate meaning	• Role-playing	• Picture boards • Puppet play/drama, etc. • Assistive technology computer programs/electronic devices

Matching visual and kinesthetic supports with verbal instruction in multiple settings will help students advance communication and formalize abstract concepts (Bellini 2006). The more students understand social situations and expectations, the better their ability to engage in diverse peer groups and develop new and appropriate relationships across a variety of settings (Bellini 2006). When students are better prepared to navigate social situations, they are also better equipped to navigate potential romantic or sexual relationships.

EMOTIONAL MANAGEMENT

In a span of just a few years, adolescents transition dramatically in almost all realms of their lives: they mature physically; their ability to analyze and reason develops; and their social relationships are redefined (Perkins and Borden 2003). The importance of emotional health in this process cannot be understated, but adolescents with IDDs and ASDs often experience deregulated emotional maintenance (Perkins and Borden 2003). These struggles can limit basic understanding of how emotion connects to thoughts and behaviors and how it ultimately affects other people's thoughts and behaviors.

"[Children with IDD and ASD] need to learn to identify and avoid situations that can lead to certain emotions, and to understand that other people have different emotions from them. Developing and learning in all of these areas, even for typically developing people, is a lifelong and difficult process" (Hartman 2014, 149).

This kind of emotional maintenance has a strong connection to sexuality. It is important to understand that any feelings of love and desirability are part of being human, whether it is as simple as a crush or as complex as experiencing feelings of homosexuality. The failure to understand and manage these emotions ultimately results in limited understanding of people and relationships, which leads to a lack of personal fulfillment.

Teaching Emotional Maintenance

There are ways to incorporate emotional maintenance in everyday practice in the classroom (table 3.4); parents and educators can help students with IDDs and ASDs to improve their emotional understanding and regulation by emphasizing five core skills:

Table 3.4   Recommendations to Help Students Build Emotional Maintenance

In order to help students . . .	*Teach this:*
Be aware of and understand feelings	• Positive and negative emotions • Privacy rules, especially when talking about sexual feelings • Body awareness to understand the physical and emotional connection in their bodies • Body's reaction to different emotions • How to identify different feelings • Preventative measures for emotional maintenance (a good night's sleep, well-balanced diet, exercising, and therapeutic supports) • The evolution of feelings, ways they can change over time
Be aware of and understand other's feelings	• The importance of learning other's feelings • The importance of expressing feelings • Strategies to ask people about their feelings • Recognizing that people can feel many emotions at the same time • Recognizing that people can show the same emotion in different ways
Express a range of emotions	• The importance of expressing feelings to other people • When and where to discuss emotions • Strategies to engage in positive self-talk • Strategies to cope with negative self-talk

In order to help students . . .	Teach this:
Express strong emotions appropriately	• How to appropriately express certain feelings • The difference between sexual and romantic feelings • Strategies to regulate emotions • Strategies for relaxation
Communicate needs and wants	• Verbal and nonverbal communicative styles • Appropriate social pragmatic skills for age, developmental stage, and environment

CONCLUSION

When teachers prioritize self-determination, social skills, and emotional maintenance, they are better able to connect with their students. The benefits are clear—when relationships are at the forefront of classroom experiences, students have opportunities to explore personal likes and dislikes and strengths and challenges, which easily lead to increased motivation, academic and behavioral engagement, and rapport among the classroom community. Allowing students to work autonomously emphasizes the enjoyment of learning relationships with peers, which contributes to self-confidence, increases student motivation, and promotes relationships in diverse settings.

RESOURCES

There are several organizations promoting awareness among parents, caregivers, and educators about the early signs of communication, speech and language skills, and social pragmatics:

• *Identify the Signs* is a campaign for early awareness, detection, and intervention. Their website: http://identifythesigns.org/.
• The *American Speech-Language-Hearing Association* (ASHA) consistently distributes information on the changing characteristics of speech and language; they provide resources for classrooms and the workplace, and offer recommendations to foster development. Their website: http://www.asha.org/public/.
• http://www.speechpathology.com/ is an ASHA-approved, paid-for resource that offers over 350 courses, live webinars, and videos for parents/caregivers, educators, and speech and language pathologists.
• The *National Association for Hearing and Speech Action* (NAHSA) supports initiatives to provide critical information for addressing

and even preventing communication problems. Their website: asha.org/NAHSA/
- *ASHA ProFind* provides an easy way for consumers to find a qualified audiologist or speech-language pathologist. Their website: asha.org/profind/

Some books that support educators, parents, and the students' social and emotional management can be purchased through the website https://www.socialthinking.com/Products. This site allows you to browse this company's approach to social and emotional skills easily by filtering choices through basic content, age of student (through adulthood), social topics, diagnosis, or by your own profession/role with the child you are servicing.

Other resources include the following online PDF:

- Promoting Self-Determination Among Students with Disabilities: A Guide for Tennessee Educators: https://vkc.mc.vanderbilt.edu/assets/files/resources/psiSelfdetermination.pdf
- Self-Monitoring Equipping Students to Manage Their Own Behavior in the Classroom: https://vkc.mc.vanderbilt.edu/assets/files/resources/psiSelfmonitoring.pdf

Additional articles for social and emotional management include the following (available from socialthinking.com):

- "Learning to Take Control of Emotional Reactions as Part of Problem Solving", by Beckham Linton and Michelle Garcia Winner.
- "Social Behavior Mapping: Connecting Behavior, Emotions, and Consequences Across the Day", by Michelle Garcia Winner.
- "Social Behavior Starts with Social Thought: The Four Steps of Perspective Taking", by Michelle Garcia Winner.

REFERENCES

American Speech-Language-Hearing Association. (2017). Retrieved November 3, 2017. http://www.asha.org/public/speech/disorders/Preschool-Language-Disorders/.

Bell, L., Magill, L., Carter, E. W., and Lane, K. L. (2013). *Self-monitoring: Equipping students to manage their own behavior in the classroom*. Project Support and Include, Vanderbilt University, Nashville, Tennessee.

Bellini, S. (2009). The development of social anxiety in adolescents with autism spectrum disorders. *Focus on Autism and Other Developmental Disabilities*, 21(3): 138–145.

Brown, F., Appel, C., Corsi, L., and Wenig, B. (1993). Choice diversity for people with severe disabilities. *Education and Training in Mental Retardation*, 28: 318–26.

Cabeza, B., Magill, L., Jenkins, A., Carter, E. W., Greiner, S., Bell, L., and Lane, K. L. (2013). *Promoting self-determination among students with disabilities: A guide for Tennessee educators*. Project Support and Include, Vanderbilt University, Nashville, Tennessee.

do2learn.com (2017). A resource for individuals with special needs. Retrieved January 25, 2018. http://www.do2learn.com.

Eyres, R., Williamson, R. L., Hunter, W., and Casey, L. (2016). Providing comprehensive sexuality education to students with intellectual and developmental disabilities: preparing the trainer. *Division on Autism and Developmental Disabilities Online Journal*, 3(1): 160–71.

Gallagher, T. (1991). (Ed.). *Pragmatics of language: Clinical practice issues*. San Diego, CA: Singular Publishing Group.

Gilliam, W. S. (2005). *Prekindergarteners left behind: Expulsion rates in state prekindergarten systems*. New Haven, CT: Yale University Child Study Center.

Hartman, D. (2014). *Sexuality and relationship education for children and adolescents with autism spectrum disorders: A professional's guide to understanding, preventing issues, supporting sexuality and responding to inappropriate behaviors*. London: Jessica Kingsley Publishers.

The Healthy Bodies Toolkit. (2013). Vanderbilt Kennedy Center. Nashville, TN.

National Parent Center on Transition and Employment. (2017). Retrieved November 3, 2017. http://www.pacer.org/transition.

Perkins, D. F., and Borden, L. M. (2003). Positive behaviors, problem behaviors, and resiliency in adolescence. In R. M. Lerner, M. A. Easterbrooks, and J. Mistry (Vol. Eds.) and I. B. Weiner (Series Ed.), *Handbook of psychology: Volume 6, Developmental psychology* (373–94). New York: Wiley.

Ryan, R. M., and Deci, E. L. (2000). Self-determination theory and the facilitation of intrinsic motivation, social development, and well-being. *American Psychologist*, 55(1): 68–78.

Taylor, R., Richards, S., and Brady, M. (2005). *Mental retardation: Historical perspectives, current practices, and future directions*. Boston: Pearson, Allyn, and Bacon.

Travers, J., Tincani, M., Whitby, P., and Boutot, A. E. (2014). Alignment of sexuality education with self-determination for people with significant disabilities: A review of research and future directions. *Education and Training in Autism and Developmental Disabilities*, 49(2): 232–47.

The United Nations. (2006). Convention on the Rights of Persons with Disabilities. *Treaty Series*, 2515: 3.

Walker-Hirsch, L. (2007). *The facts of life . . . and more: Sexuality and intimacy for people with intellectual disabilities*. Baltimore, MD: Paul H. Brooks Publishing.

Wehmeyer, M. L. (2007). *Promoting self-determination in students with developmental disabilities*. New York: Guilford Press.

Wehmeyer, M. L., and Field, S. (2007). *Self-determination: Instructional and assessment strategies*. Thousand Oaks, CA: Corwin Press.

Wehmeyer, M. L., and Palmer, S. B. (2003). Adult outcomes for students with cognitive disabilities three-years after high school: The impact of self-determination. *Education and Training in Developmental Disabilities*, 38(2): 131–44.

Wilkenfeld, B. F., and Ballan, M. S. (2011). Educators' attitudes and beliefs towards the sexuality of individuals with developmental disabilities. *Sexuality and Disability*, 29: 351–61.

Chapter 4

We Can't Hide:
Pop Culture and Digital Media

I've had tons of bullies who would call me retarded, even on my Facebook page. It's sad and it really hurts. I want to tell people not to use the word. Don't say your friend's retarded when they do something foolish.

—Lauren Potter, advocate for disability rights and award-winning actress with Down syndrome; best known for playing the role of cheerleader Becky Jackson on the hit TV show *Glee*

SUMMARY

Entertainment media can be an avenue for promoting accurate information for and about people with intellectual disabilities and autism. However, stereotypes and misleading, inaccurate portrayals are common. Individuals with disabilities are rarely depicted in romantic relationships or as having social connections. Digital media offers the opportunity for social interaction and intimate relationships, but for those with IDDs and ASDs, its use can also result in misinterpretations and negative social and emotional consequences. After reading this chapter, readers will be able to identify (see Figure 1):

- the negative effects of pejorative language used to describe individuals with intellectual disabilities and the use of respectful, humanistic language;
- the principles of person-first philosophy and identity-first language;
- the positive and negative ways people with intellectual or developmental disabilities (IDDs) and autism spectrum disorders (ASDs) are portrayed in popular culture and ways to dispel stereotypes;

- possible consequences, both positive and negative, for people with IDDs and ASDs when accessing the Internet and using social media;
- teaching tools and interventions for educators, parents, and counselors to improve understanding of the benefits and risks of using digital media for individuals with IDDs and ASDs.

STEREOTYPES IN ENTERTAINMENT MEDIA

When people with disabilities are depicted in literature, movies, television, and news, they typically fall into predictable categories: tragic heroes with almost superhuman qualities who overcome obstacles in spite of their disabilities, appealing, yet pitiful, victims who often possess childlike qualities, or evil villains who turn to crime due to resentment over their disabilities (Lester and Ross 2003). These stereotypes may seem like harmless entertainment, but, in fact, when people do not have direct contact with individuals with disabilities, they are likely to form opinions based on what they read about, see, or hear in popular media. Table 4.1 describes these stereotypes.

To make matters worse, people with IDDs and ASDs have been historically underrepresented in entertainment media, and when they do appear, the characters are often based on negative stereotypes that are stigmatizing and present inaccurate messages. Actors frequently give exaggerated performances displaying every possible symptom from the diagnostic criteria of a given disability or characters are portrayed as one-dimensional and uncomplicated, often to support the storyline of a major character.

Rarely do storylines involve sexual or romantic relationships. Storylines tend to focus on the disability, rather than the individual (Barnes 1992; Lester and Ross 2003). Not only does this create an unrealistic picture of

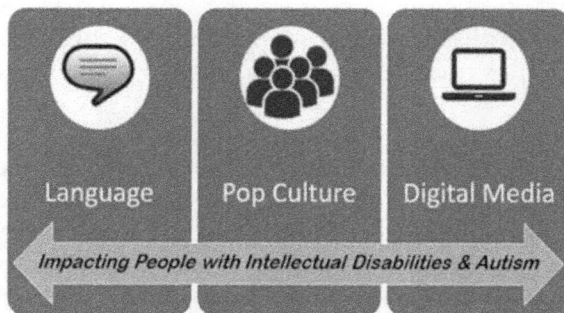

Figure 4.1   Language, Pop Culture, and Digital Media

people with disabilities, it dehumanizes by failing to portray individuals with unique feelings, thoughts, and personalities.

Common Media Stereotypes

Table 4.1   **Common Media Stereotypes**

Stereotype	Characteristics	Barriers created
Hero	• Possession of a rare talent • Superhuman power	• Creates unrealistic expectations • Minimizes the real struggles that people with disabilities face daily • Implies that a person with disability must overcome the disability or perform extraordinary acts
Victim	• Helpless • Vulnerable • Pitiful • Asexual • Childlike innocence • "A child trapped in an adult's body."	• Disempowers and objectifies people with disabilities by implying that they must be cared for and protected • Restricts age-appropriate activities • Influences caregivers to deny or remain unaware of sexual development, interests, and needs • Influences caregivers to become overprotective and to prevent access to outlets for sexual behaviors or conversation (Attwood, Henaut and Dubin, 2014)
Villain	• Less frequently used to depict individuals with IDDs and ASDs • More often used to depict physical disabilities (Lester and Ross, 2003)	• Dehumanizes individuals with disabilities • Implies that they turn to revenge out of resentment of their condition. • Implies a tendency toward criminal behavior • Creates fear of people with disabilities

Combatting Stereotypes through Language

Labels are powerful; they can be valuable tools that open doors to services and funding or weapons that create stigma and pain. Throughout history, people with IDDs and ASDs have been known by many labels. When viewed through today's lens, some sound appalling. Words like *moron* and *imbecile* were originally used by medical professionals to describe people with IDDs but took on different connotations as they entered the popular culture of the time. When they became derogatory, they were replaced by nonoffensive terms, which, in turn, took on new meanings as they filtered into society. The term *mental retardation* was adopted in the late nineteenth century and eventually developed a negative connotation, particularly as the derivative "retard" became part of the vernacular in the mid-twentieth century.

In 2009, a movement was created called "Spread the Word to End the Word" in an attempt to eradicate use of the term "retarded", which became known in some circles as "the R-word" (Reynolds, Zupanick, and Donbeck 2013). In 2010, Congress passed Rosa's Law, which changed the term "mental retardation" to "intellectual disability" and references to "a mentally retarded individual" to "an individual with an intellectual disability" in federal health, education, and labor laws and policy. Changes were also made in the *DSM-5* and public education terminology (American Psychiatric Association 2013; Reynolds et al. 2013).

Those changes are part of a larger movement among advocates and self-advocates to destigmatize and humanize people with disabilities through the use of language. "Person-first language" began in the 1980s as a way of speaking and acting that avoids sensationalizing, victimizing, or otherwise stereotyping a person because he or she has a disability ("People-first language" 2017).

EXAMPLES AND NONEXAMPLES
OF PERSON-FIRST TERMINOLOGY

An important aspect of person-first language is the practice of putting the person first and the disability second when speaking or writing. This avoids using the disability to define the person. For example, instead of saying "the disabled child," when using person-first language, one would say, "The child with a disability." Table 4.2 provides examples of person first terminology.

It is important to note that many individuals with disabilities, particularly those who are members of the deaf and blind communities, view their differences as a part of their identity and prefer not to use person-first terminology. A significant number of individuals with autism fall into this category. They embrace their differences and their labels and advocate use of "identity-first language".

Table 4.2   Person-First Terminology

Person-first terminology	Terminology to avoid
• He has Down syndrome.	• He is afflicted with Down syndrome.
• She has muscular dystrophy.	• She is a victim of muscular dystrophy.
• He uses a wheelchair.	• He is confined to a wheelchair or is wheelchair-bound.
• She is a competitor.	• She bravely competes despite her disability.
• He has autism.	• He is autistic.

The major difference between person-first and identity-first language is in how each describes an individual with a disability. For example, users of identity-first language will say "autistic person" or "deaf person" instead of "person with autism" or "person with a hearing impairment." The idea being that "autistic" and "deaf" are characteristics that are part of one's identity like race, religion, or nationality and not something negative (Dunn and Andrews 2015).

A growing number of advocacy groups and individuals strongly support identity-first language when speaking about autism. There is even a world-wide campaign called *Identity-First Autistic* that endorses the use of identity-first language. To learn more about the identity-first movement in the autistic community, visit https://www.identityfirstautistic.org/.

Another issue involving language is the label used to identify those on the higher end of the autism spectrum. Although the term *Asperger's syndrome* is no longer used as a diagnosis, it is alive and well in the autistic community. Many autism-advocacy groups continue to use terms related to Asperger in their names, mission statements, goals, and policies. People diagnosed with Asperger's syndrome can retain that label if the diagnosis was made prior to 2013, when the *DSM-5* eliminated the term. Many who have chosen to do so proudly call themselves *aspies*, a derivative of Asperger.

There is a lot of controversy among and within disability groups about whether person-first or identity-first language is appropriate. The goals of both are to promote a view of people with disabilities as individuals who have the right to be treated and spoken of with respect and dignity. There is no one way of speaking that is correct, but organizations like the Arc of the United States, Special Olympics, and the American Psychiatric Association currently advocate the use of person-first language, and most schools expect teachers and related service providers to use person-first language.

Individual preferences of the person in question should be the determining factor in deciding how one speaks about him or her. Using language that respects the individual being discussed or referred to is one of the first steps in combatting stereotypes and promoting respect for people with disabilities.

Despite the widespread push to embrace respectful language and eliminate the use of the word *retarded*, these are new concepts for many in the United States. A Harris poll (2017) found about 40 percent of adults stated they saw nothing wrong in using the word to describe a thing or situation and 50 percent have heard someone with an intellectual disability called a *retard*.

Combatting Stereotypes through Entertainment Media

Like spoken language, entertainment media has the power to influence society's perception of groups of people in a positive or a negative way. While much progress has been made to improve portrayals, a segment of entertainment media continues to perpetuate stereotypes and stigmatize people with disabilities. For example, in 2008 the movie *Tropic Thunder* received negative attention for insensitive content directed at people with intellectual disabilities and for repeated use of the word *retard*. A coalition of twenty-two advocacy groups, including the Special Olympics, the Arc of the United States, and the National Down Syndrome Congress, reacted by launching a nationwide boycott of the film (Zeidler 2008). In spite of the negative attention the film garnered, it achieved box-office success and earned almost $200 million worldwide (*Tropic Thunder*, 2008).

While there have been some notable exceptions like Lauren Potter, most characters with disabilities are played by actors without disabilities (Woodburn and Kopic 2016). Advocacy organizations like the Special Olympics continue to urge popular media to develop realistic characters with disabilities living successful lives and suggest that people with disabilities be included in story development. It appears as though some in the entertainment industry have been listening and share those feelings.

By the 2010s, more believable multidimensional characters began appearing in dramas and comedies in motion pictures and television, sometimes in title roles, and portrayals seem to be moving away from the stereotypical hero or victim. Successful movies like *The Accountant,* starring Ben Affleck, and *Extremely Loud and Incredibly Close*, with Tom Hanks, feature characters with autism in leading roles.

Several notable programs developed for the small screen also include complex characters with IDDs and ASDs. NBC's *Parenthood* sensitively addressed issues of parenting a child with autism. Lauren Potter's character, Becky, was a regular on the TV series *Glee* for six seasons. Becky was a cheerleader who also had Down syndrome. Her romantic feelings were realistically portrayed when she unsuccessfully tried to win the affection of another character.

Sheldon Cooper of CBS's long-running sitcom *The Big Bang Theory* is one of the most well-known characters on television. The series centers on four socially awkward scientists, their friendship, and their friends. Sheldon has long been assumed by many to be on the autism spectrum, but the writers have never affirmed the speculation. He has a girlfriend and their unconventional, slow-moving romantic and sexual relationship is an important, ongoing storyline.

Documentary feature films have also done a great deal to break stereotypes and raise awareness for individuals with autism and intellectual disabilities. *Autism in Love* (2015) is a PBS Independent Lens film chronicling the lives of four adults, all on the autism spectrum, and the challenges they face as they search for love and intimacy (Fuller 2016). *Life Animated* (2016), a documentary by Roger Ross Williams, follows a young adult with autism, as he uses Disney's animated movies to help him navigate socially in the world. *Monica and David* (2009), an HBO documentary film, follows a newly married couple with Down syndrome through their first year of marriage.

All three films have received positive reviews from advocacy groups and are sold as educational DVDs with public performance rights. They provide opportunities for discussion of the complex issues of intimacy, marriage, sex, loss, and love for individuals with ASDs and IDDs, and their teachers, counselors, and families. These films also showcase the unique ways in which the disabilities affect the lives of the stars, while depicting them as people first. Their challenges and celebrations are ones that an average person can relate to; they are realistic, emotional, and honest.

While there is controversy surrounding the ethics and accuracy of so-called reality TV, it is this genre that portrays the most characters with disabilities and employs the greatest number of actors with disabilities (Kidd 2014). At its worst, reality TV exploits its stars and sensationalizes disabilities, but at its best, it challenges damaging stereotypes and promotes meaningful discussion by presenting a "normalized" view of the lives of people with disabilities.

For example, *Born This Way* is a reality TV series on the A&E cable network that entered its third season in 2017. It follows the lives of seven young adults with Down syndrome and their parents as they react and adjust to challenges and successes in their everyday lives. The show addresses issues such as dating, sex, health care, and self-determination. *Born This Way* has been well received by many disability advocates. Randy Rutta (2016), the CEO of Easter Seals, said this about the program:

> *Born This Way* set out to change the way the world views young adults with disabilities and their potential—looking beyond the disability and focusing on the person: a son, daughter, friend, sibling, girlfriend, boyfriend or fiancé. . . . Millennials living with disabilities, those who grew up with the ADA, have high expectations for their future. They want and deserve careers and independence. All they need is opportunity. And it starts with taking on the stigma. Taking on the inequality. Taking on the challenges that people with disabilities and the disability community face across myriad issues and the landscape of American society.

Easter Seals blogger Erin Hawley (2016) provides a counterpoint with these words of caution regarding reality TV programs that feature people with disabilities:

> I want us included in media, and I am not opposed to reality shows starring people with disabilities on their own terms. Yet a part of me wonders if others are watching just because they can stare at us from the comfort of their couch.

In person, people tend to steal glances at me when they think I am not looking or won't notice. There is a long, problematic history of exploitation and people with disabilities masked as entertainment (think carnivals), and I question whether or not these reality TV shows might be the modern extension of that.

Regardless of motives of the audience and the producers, documentaries on both the big and small screen have a large viewership and have done much to provide a more accurate look at multidimensional people with disabilities in real-world scenarios involving love, romance, and sexual relationships.

The early part of the twenty-first century saw some important firsts that have broken barriers for people with IDDs and ASDs in American pop culture. Women with autism and Down syndrome have competed in the Miss America and Miss USA beauty pageants (Blanchette 2017; Oldenburg 2013). In 2007, when a contestant with Asperger's syndrome finished in fourth place on the hit TV series *America's Next Top Model,* the subject of females with autism became a topic of discussion in the media (Parker-Popedek 2007).

In 2015, Jamie Brewer, best known for her roles in the FX TV series *American Horror Story,* became the first person with Down syndrome to walk the red carpet at New York's Fashion week (Jamie Brewer, n.d.). Perhaps the most promising development for changing society's attitudes comes from the children's TV series *Sesame Street.* As part of its autism initiative, *Sesame Street and Autism: See Amazing in All Children,* the character of Julia, a Muppet with autism, debuted in 2016 (*Sesame Street* 2017).

Individuals' Use of Digital Media: Risks and Rewards

A popular misconception involving people with IDDs and ASDs is that they are uninterested in forming friendships or romantic relationships and, in the case of those with ASD, prefer being alone. In fact, many feel the pain of loneliness and long for meaningful relationships but lack the skills and understanding needed to keep and maintain relationships, and lack the opportunities to meet and socialize with others in a romantic or sexual way (Bauminger and Kasari 2000; Mazurek 2014).

Most people with ASDs and IDDs, like their typical peers, want to date and often turn to the Internet to help them understand and be successful in romantic and sexual relationships. As with typical peers, online dating is gaining in popularity (Roth and Gillis 2015). Digital technology has become a vital part of today's culture. Smartphones and tablets are considered necessities by many people and are important tools that can help level the social playing field for those with disabilities. People with IDDs and ASDs often access the Internet regularly and do it most often with a smartphone or tablet (Chadwick, Wesson, and Fullwood 2013). Many have grown up with and view their computer as a familiar comfortable way to gather information and often as a primary source of entertainment. Table 4.3 provides ideas about topics for instruction for internet safety.

Digital media represents a myriad of possibilities to expand social capital for people with ASDs and IDDs, creating new opportunities to interact and communicate with others via e-mail and text, voice, or video chats. There is convincing evidence that using social media can improve social interactions, reduce feelings of loneliness, and provide a sense of well-being for users with disabilities (Chadwick et al. 2013; Shpigelman 2016).

There are obvious benefits for people who struggle with the fast-paced, give-and-take exchanges that make up typical conversations. The ability to make inferences and understand nonverbal language in face-to-face communication is difficult, if not impossible for some with ASDs and IDDs, and can cause anxiety, which, in turn, can increase the likelihood of misunderstandings, communication lapses, and social faux pas (Roth and Gillis 2015). Texting and computer-mediated communication have the potential to eliminate some of those problems. Voice or video chats can provide an option for communication for those who have trouble typing and reading.

Digital devices and Internet access can serve as valuable tools for individuals with IDDs and ASDs who want to learn about, start, and maintain emotional and physical relationships, but they also pose significant threats that should not be ignored (Attwood et al. 2014; Chadwick et al. 2013). Due to deficits in understanding social cues, communication styles, and theory of mind, they may not realize that they are being taken advantage of or made fun of online.

Stalking and harassment are possible problem behaviors that can result from lack of understanding of social media and texting etiquette (Attwood et al. 2017; Baker 2013; Roth and Gillis 2015). They may not understand the difference between flirtatious and threatening language and may not realize that people they meet online could be projecting a false identity. Instructing adolescents and adults on the law regarding child pornography and the dangers to both personal and professional relationships of posting explicit pictures and text is essential (Attwood et al. 2017; Baker 2013).

Furthermore, they should understand how to avoid being the victim or perpetrator in any of those activities and what to do if they realize that they have become the victim or the perpetrator. Rules about cyberbullying, e-mailing, accessing the Internet, and viewing online pornography while at work or school should be explicitly taught. Evidence-based social skills programs and teacher-created lessons that include direct instruction, modeling, role-playing, practicing the skill in different settings, and performance feedback can be used to teach some of these skills.

The use of games, Social Stories®, comic book conversations, and natural environment teaching is also effective (Attwood et al. 2014). The five-point scale, developed by Kari Dunn Buron, is especially useful in making the abstract ideas surrounding use of the Internet and social media into visual, concrete rules or guidelines (Buron 2007).

While it is far more common for individuals with disabilities to be victims of sex crimes, there is a real danger for individuals with autism and IDDs to intentionally or unintentionally interact with illegal pornography (Attwood et al. 2014). In his book *No More Victims* (2013), Jed Baker uses the popular Internet meme *Rule 34*, "If it exists, someone has made porn out of it. No exceptions," to illustrate that even with filters, pornography is easy to access. Google and YouTube searches for characters from television series, cartoons, and video games that are popular with children can lead to pornographic or violent videos and images.

The case of Nick Dubin can serve as a cautionary tale of the dangers that exist for people who do not understand the law, social cues, and theory of mind, and are not able to recognize dangerous situations. Nick Dubin is a successful writer and was well known as an advocate for people on the autism spectrum. He appeared to be well grounded and confident. However, he was socially isolated and bullied for most of his life and was not diagnosed with Asperger's syndrome until the age of 27.

Assessment of Nick's adaptive skills revealed scores in the preadolescent level. He was not sexually active and also lacked basic information about sexuality. Failing to understand the moral, ethical, and legal rules associated with child pornography, Nick downloaded child pornography through the Internet. As a result of this naive action, Nick was arrested and convicted on a felony count of possession of child pornography. In his book *The Autism Spectrum, Sexuality and the Law*, Nick writes:

> After I was arrested, my therapist explained to me that the children in the images I was viewing are victims and I feel great remorse for their degradation. Unfortunately, I was not able to make these connections prior to my arrest and I deeply regret my actions. My greatest sadness is wishing that I knew then what I know now. (Attwood et al. 2014)

The vulnerability of males on the autism spectrum regarding child pornography is controversial. When Eustacia Cutler, well-known author and speaker and mother of Temple Grandin, wrote in the *Daily Beast* (2013) about this "toxic combination," she received a great deal of criticism from many advocates who viewed her comments as baseless and damaging. In response to the controversy Culter's article generated, John Elder Robison (2013), a writer and advocate who also has autism, wrote:

> This situation is particularly tragic because technology has made it so easy to commit a sex crime. A $20 webcam becomes an instrument of a felony, as does

the keyboard of an iPad. It's a reality many middle-aged parents and teachers overlook because this sort of thing simply wasn't possible when we ourselves were young. . . . Some know it's wrong, and go down the path anyway. Others don't really understand what they are doing. Few of these people are truly threats to the public, yet all end up in terrible trouble when they run up against the law.

But I do feel our differences can place us at risk in some situations and this is one of them.

What do you think? *Cutler did not cite any statistics to support the idea that men with ASD are more likely to view child pornography. In fact, little quantitative data exists. Was she perpetuating the villain stereotype, or was she shedding light on a real problem?*

Table 4.3   Suggested Topics for Instruction in Internet Safety

• Risks and consequences of posting explicit images and messages online	• How to recognize and report cyberbullying and cyberstalking
• Differences between legal and illegal pornography and the dangers both pose	• Specific language to use and avoid in online conversations
• Acceptable and nonacceptable images to share via online posts or texts	• E-mail policies of possible employers
• Understanding privacy settings and why they are important	• Rules about when and how often to text
• How to safely create a personal profile	• Differences between an online friend and a real-life friend
• Risks and consequences of posting messages and images impulsively when hurt or angry	• The meaning of common terms used in social media
• Cyberstalking vs. online flirting	• Clues that an online friend may be using a false identity
	• How to unfriend someone on Facebook

SCENARIOS FOR DISCUSSION

What do you think? *Read and reflect on each of the following scenarios. How would you intervene with each of the individuals? What topics would you teach, and how would you teach them?*

Scenario One: A high school graduate experiences the isolation that many feel when they no longer have access to the social group that school provides. He befriends and, without telling friends or family, travels out of state to spend a weekend with an older man he met online. When he returns, he posts pictures of gay pornography on his Facebook page and is quickly unfriended by most of his high school friends.

Scenario Two: A high school couple with IDD has a volatile on-again/off-again relationship. During one breakup, the boy posts intimate photos of the girl, with derogatory comments. Although they are only a year apart in age, the girl is a minor, but the boy is not. He is guilty of posting illegal pornography.

Scenario Three: In a quest to start romantic relationships, a young man repeatedly texts several girls' pictures of small spaces and asks if they can fit into them. It is difficult to convince him to stop, since the perseverative behavior and lack of social cognition make it difficult for him to perceive the damage he is doing to his reputation and the harm he is doing to the very people from whom he seeks acceptance. He becomes well known and is avoided for his bizarre, unwanted behavior.

Scenario Four: A young adult blogger with ASD who has not disclosed his disability uses his professional site to vent his frustrations about not being able to find a girlfriend or have an intimate relationship. He shares personal information and makes graphic statements describing his despair and self-loathing. He loses many followers and a job for which he was being considered.

CONCLUSION

When negative, inaccurate stereotypes of people with disabilities are perpetuated in popular culture, much damage is done to the quality of life of the individuals who are targeted.

RESOURCES

Internet Resources

- *eBuddies* is a division of Best Buddies for people with and without IDDs to come together online to form friendships: bestbuddies.org
- *Spread the Word to End the Word* offers many resources for raising awareness, including activities, fact sheets, and information on why it is important to stop using hurtful speech and how you or your group can help: www.r-word.org

Books/Articles and Other Resources

- *No More Victims* by Jed Baker is a small book packed with ideas for instruction in Internet safety, written for individuals with ASDs but suitable for all learners.
- *Digital Citizenship Program from Common Sense Standard* aligned lesson plans by grade and subject, with videos, essential questions, and activities.

Topics include Internet safety, cyberbullying, relationships, and more. Common Sense is an independent nonprofit organization that provides high-quality digital literacy and citizenship programs to educators and school communities (commonsense.org/education/digital-citizenship).

How to Stay Current on the Subject:

- Subscribe to *Disability Scoop*—the nation's largest news organization devoted to coverage of developmental disabilities: disabilityscoop.com
- Connect with your local chapter of Best Buddies, the Arc, and Special Olympics.

REFERENCES

American Psychiatric Association. (2013). *Diagnostic and statistical manual of mental disorders: DSM-5*. Washington, DC: American Psychiatric Association.

Attwood, T., Henaut, I., and Dubin, N. A. (2014). *The autism spectrum, sexuality and the law*. London, England: Jessica Kingsley Publishers.

Baker, J. (2013). *No more victims: Protecting those with autism from cyberbullying, internet predators and scams*. Arlington, TX: Future Horizons, Inc.

Barnes, C. (1992) *Disabling imagery and the media: An exploration of the principles for media representations of disabled people*. Krumlin, Halifax, England: The British Council of Organisations of Disabled People and Ryburn Publishing Limited.

Bauminger, N., and Kasari, C. (2000). Loneliness and friendship in high-functioning children with autism. *Child Development*, 71: 2.

Blanchette, A. (2017, April 22). Woman with Down syndrome to compete in Miss Minnesota USA pageant. *Minneapolis Star Tribune*. http://www.startribune.com/first-woman-with-down-syndrome-to-compete-in-miss-minnesota-usa-pageant/420145783/.

Buron, K. (2007). *A 5 is against the law! Social boundaries: Straight up! An honest guide for teens and young adults*. Shawnee Mission, KS: Autism Asperger Publishing Company.

Chadwick, D., Wesson, C., and Fullwood, C. (2013). Internet access by people with intellectual disabilities: Inequalities and opportunities. *Future Internet*, 5(3): 376–397.

Cutler, E. (2013). Autism and child pornography: A toxic combination: Why autistic men are viewing child pornography—and being labeled sex offenders. *Daily Beast*. http://www.thedailybeast.com/autism-and-child-pornography-a-toxic-combination.

Dunn, S., and Andrews, E. (2015). Person-first and identity-first language: Developing psychologists' cultural competence using disability language. *American Psychologist*, 70: 3.

Fuller, M. (2016). *Autism in love*. http://www.pbs.org/independentlens/films/autism-in-love/.

Haller, B., and Zhang, L. (2014). Stigma or empowerment? What do disabled people say about their representation in news and entertainment media? *Review of Disability Studies*, 9: 4.

Harris Poll. (2017). *R-Word* (Data file). http://media.theharrispoll.com/documents/HarrisPoll_RWord_CompleteResults.pdf.

Hawley, E. (2016, March 9). Disability representation on reality television is a complicated issue [Web log comment]. http://blog.easterseals.com/disability-representation-on-reality-television-is-a-complicated-issue/.

Jamie Brewer. (n.d.). In IMDb, the Internet movie database. Retrieved June 10, 2017. http://www.imdb.com/name/nm4661932/bio?ref_=nm_ov_bio_sm.

Kidd, D. (2014) *Pop culture freaks: Identity, mass media, and society*. Boulder, CO: Westview Press.

Lester, P., and Ross, S. (2003). *Images that injure: Pictorial stereotypes in the media* (2nd ed.). Westport, CT: Greenwood Publishing Group. Mazurek, M. (2014). Loneliness, friendship, and well-being in adults with autism spectrum disorders. *Autism,* 18(3): 223–32. https://doi.org/10.1177/1362361312474121.

Monica and David. (n.d.). Retrieved November 3, 2017. http://www.monicaanddavid.com/.

Oldenburg, A. (2013, January 11). Miss Montana: First autistic Miss America contestant. *USA Today*. https://www.usatoday.com/story/life/people/2013/01/11/miss-montana-first-autistic-miss-america-contestant/1827539/.

Parker-Popedek, T. (2007, December 4). Asperger's syndrome gets a very public face. *New York Times*. http://www.nytimes.com/2007/12/04/health/04well.html.

"People First language." (2017, July 11). In *WordSense.eu online dictionary*. http://www.wordsense.eu/people-first_language.

Reynolds, T., Zupanick, C., and Donbeck, M. (2013). History of stigmatizing names for intellectual disabilities continued. https://www.mentalhelp.net/articles/history-of-stigmatizing-names-for-intellectual-disabilities-continued/.

Robison, J. (2013, August 6). Autism and porn: A problem no one talks about. Are people with autism more vulnerable to the lure of pornography? [Web log comment]. http://blog.easterseals.com/entertainment-thats-helping-society-gain-new-perspective-on-disability/.

Roth, M., and Gillis, J. (2015). Convenience with the click of a mouse: A survey of adults with autism spectrum disorder on online dating. *Sexuality and Disability*, 33: 1.

Rutta, R. (2016, July 26). Entertainment that's helping society gain new perspective on disability [Web log comment]. http://blog.easterseals.com/entertainment-thats-helping-society-gain-new-perspective-on-disability/.

Sesame Street and autism: See amazing in all children. (2017). http://autism.sesamestreet.org.

Shpigelman, C. N. (2016, December 21). Leveraging social capital of individuals with intellectual disabilities through participation in facebook. *Journal of Applied Research in Intellectual Disabilities*.

Shpigelman, C. N., and Gill, C. J. (2014). How do adults with intellectual disabilities use Facebook? *Disability and Society,* 29(10): 610–625. DOI: 10.1080/09687599.2 014.966186.

Tropic thunder. (2008). In IMDb, the internet movie database. Retrieved from http:// www.imdb.com/title/tt0942385/.

Woodburn, D., and Kopic, K. (2016). *The Ruderman white paper on employment of actors with disabilities in television* [White paper]. Retrieved November 3, 2017. http://www.rudermanfoundation.org/blog/article/the-ruderman-white-paper-employment-of-actors-with-disabilities-in-television.

Zeidler, S. (2008, August 11). Advocates for disabled to protest "Tropic Thunder." http://www.reuters.com/article/us-boycott-disability-idUSN1029346220080811.

Chapter 5

The Birds and the Bees, Round 2: The Curriculum

Comprehensive life skills-based sexuality education helps young people to gain the knowledge and skills to make conscious, healthy and respectful choices about relationships and sexuality.

—United Nations Educational, Scientific, and Cultural Organization, 2015.

Sexuality education is a life-long process of acquiring information and forming attitudes, beliefs, and values.

— SIECUS, 2004.

SUMMARY

Sexuality education programs that comprehensively teach critical thinking skills regarding human sexuality foster safer sexual practices and delayed sexual activity. In contrast, abstinence-only programs have not proven effective in reducing teen pregnancies or sexually transmitted diseases (United Nations Educational, Scientific and Cultural Organization 2015). A need exists for all young people, with and without intellectual disabilities, to have access to comprehensive sexuality education (CSE).

Topics recommended by the American Academy of Pediatrics (Breuner and Mattson 2016) include intimate relationships, human sexual anatomy, sexual reproduction, sexually transmitted infections, sexual activity, sexual orientation, gender identity, abstinence, contraception, and reproductive rights and responsibilities. After reading this chapter, readers will understand:

- the history of sexuality and relationship education and persons with intellectual or developmental disabilities (IDDs) and on the autism spectrum
  disorders (ASDs);
- comprehensive sexuality education definition, components, and evaluation;
- persons with IDDs and ASDs and sexual offenses;
- evidence-informed and data-driven theory, lessons, and practice;
- transition planning; and
- current sexuality and relationship education programs designed for persons
  with IDDs and ASDs.

THE HISTORY OF SEXUALITY AND RELATIONSHIP EDUCATION AND PERSONS WITH IDDS

The topic of sexuality and relationship education and people with IDDs and
ASDs is a sensitive one for many people. Throughout history, there has been
little effort to create a meaningful curriculum to provide appropriate information on sexuality and relationships for people with IDDs and ASDs. People
with intellectual disabilities were often viewed as having an incomplete or
underdeveloped adulthood. Subsequently, they were considered asexual persons and infantilized.

This attitude, along with concern for "racial hygiene," led to the widespread practice of eugenics beginning in the early 1900s. Eugenics is the
uninformed or nonconsensual sterilization of people with IDDs and ASDs,
and continued until the 1980s (Gougeon 2009). Although eugenics largely
ended in the 1980s, the widespread use of contraception for people with
IDDs and ASDs continues to this day, due, in part, to the fact that sex education for people with IDDs and ASDs has historically been incomplete to
nonexistent.

Formal sexuality education for people with IDDs and ASDs has tended
to be reactive, initiated by caregivers and educators after students become
sexually active, rather than proactive, providing information before students
become sexually active. The sexuality education provided to people with
IDDs and ASDs is often either vague or euphemistic (i.e., birds and bees)
or overly technical, stressing functional sexuality over pleasure and relationships (Gougeon 2009).

In addition to the lack of formal sexual education, people with IDDs and
ASDs often miss out on the typical informal education adolescents get outside the classroom. This information, correct or incorrect, forms a significant
portion of what Gougeon refers to as the "ignored curriculum."

COMPREHENSIVE SEXUALITY EDUCATION DEFINITION AND COMPONENTS

Comprehensive sexuality education (CSE) goes far beyond the topic of sexual behavior and encompasses key components as outlined by the Sexuality Information and Education Council of the United States (SIECUS, 2004) and the American Academy of Pediatrics (AAP; 2016). CSE uses ongoing developmentally appropriate, age-respective, and evidence-based education about sexuality, sexual reproduction, relationships, and sexual health provided by pediatricians, educators, other professionals, and parents (Breuner and Mattson 2016).

CSE is not a one-time class; rather, it is a lifespan process providing in-depth information, which can equip youth in making informed, positive, and safe choices about relationships, sexual activity, and sexual health (SIECUS, 2004). The key components recommended by these two organizations are listed in table 5.1. Box 5.1 provides the comprehensive plan for sexuality education.

These components provide context for ensuring CSE spans intimate relationships, human sexual anatomy, sexual reproduction, and developmentally appropriate sexual health–related knowledge, attitudes, skills, and practices. Qualified, trained teachers should provide sexuality education on sexually transmitted infections (STIs), sexual activity, consent, sexual orientation, abstinence, contraception, and reproductive rights and responsibilities.

National Sexuality Education Standards

The Future of Sex Education (FoSE) project (2007) promotes CSE in all K–12 schools of United States with a vision of healthy sexual development for all students. The first-ever National Sexuality Education Standards for

Table 5.1   Key Components of Comprehensive Sexuality Education

SIECUS	AAP
– Human development	– Healthy sexual development
– Relationships	– Gender identity
– Personal skills	– Interpersonal relationships
– Sexual behavior	– Affection
– Sexual health	– Intimacy
– Society and culture	– Body image

BOX 5.1   COMPREHENSIVE SEXUALITY EDUCATION

A planned, sequential K–12 curriculum that is part of a comprehensive school health education approach addresses age-appropriate physical, mental, emotional, and social dimensions of human sexuality. The curriculum should be designed to motivate and assist students to maintain and improve their sexual health, prevent disease, and reduce sexual health–related risk behaviors. It should allow students to develop and demonstrate developmentally appropriate sexual health–related knowledge, attitudes, skills, and practices. The comprehensive sexuality education curriculum should include a variety of topics including anatomy, physiology, families, personal safety, healthy relationships, pregnancy and birth, sexually transmitted diseases including HIV, contraceptives, sexual orientation, pregnancy options, media literacy, and more. It should be medically accurate. Qualified, trained teachers should provide sexuality education.

(Future of Sex Education 2012; http://www.futureofsexed.org/resources.html)

---

school-age children was made available in 2012 (Future of Sex Education Initiative 2012) to support educators in working toward this vision. The sequential K–12 curriculum standards (figure 5.1) outline for educators what to teach and how to teach.

LACK OF EDUCATOR TRAINING

Typically, educators are not provided training in school to address the sexual health needs of students. Lack of exposure to the content and feeling inadequately prepared to teach sexuality education results in many educators avoiding the topic for students—especially students with IDDs and ASDs (Aunos and Feldman 2002; Barnard-Brak, Schmidt, Chesnut, Wei, and Richman 2014; Howard-Barr et al. 2005). To address this need of teacher training/preparation, FoSE developed the *National Teacher Preparation Standards for Sexuality Education* (Barr et al. 2014). Figure 5.1 presents the sequence of K–12 standards relating to sexuality education, the standards are summarized in figure 5.2.

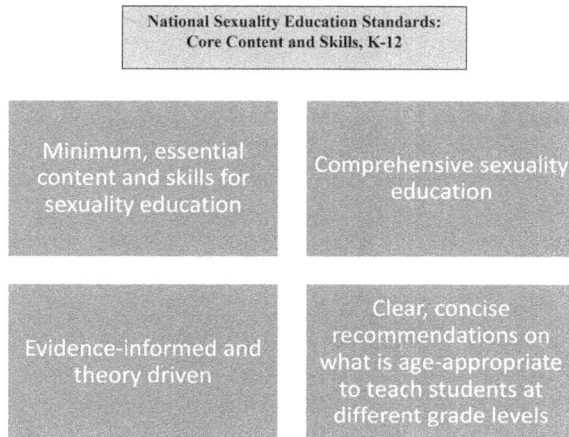

National Sexuality Education Standards:
Core Content and Skills, K-12

Minimum, essential content and skills for sexuality education

Comprehensive sexuality education

Evidence-informed and theory driven

Clear, concise recommendations on what is age-appropriate to teach students at different grade levels

Figure 5.1   Sequential K–12 Curriculum Standards

Standard 1: Professional Disposition Teacher candidates demonstrate comfort with, commitment to, and self-efficacy in teaching sexuality education.

Standard 2: Diversity and Equity Teacher candidates show respect for individual, family and cultural characteristics and experiences that may influence student learning about sexuality.

Standard 3: Content Knowledge Teacher candidates have accurate and current knowledge of the biological, emotional, social, and legal aspects of human sexuality.

Standard 4: Legal and Professional Ethics Teacher candidates make decisions based on applicable federal, state and local laws, regulations and policies, as well as professional ethics.

Standard 5: Planning Teacher candidates plan age- and developmentally appropriate sexuality education that is aligned with standards, policies, and laws and reflects the diversity of the community.

Standard 6: Implementation Teacher candidates use a variety of effective strategies to teach sexuality education.

Standard 7: Assessment Teacher candidates implement effective strategies to assess student knowledge, attitudes, and skills in order to improve sexuality education instruction.

Figure 5.2   National Teacher Preparation Standards for Sexuality Education.
Adapted from National Teacher Preparation Standards for Sexuality Education.

PARENTS/FAMILIES AS EDUCATORS
OF SEXUALITY INFORMATION

Parents and caregivers share an important role in teaching their children about sexual health topics. Ideally, they provide the primary sexuality education in relation to familial values and culture/religious social norms specific to intimate, sexual relationships (Shtarkshall, Santelli, and Hirsch 2007). Parents and caregivers, however, are often not equipped to provide CSE, so collaboration with educators can foster open dialogue with school staff and family.

Currently, limited research exists on engaging parents in sexuality education alongside educators. Further investigation into parental roles may also help identify resistance CSE and how communication, training, and awareness can lead to more effective program implementation.

Training/Awareness for Parents/Family and Educators

More research is also needed to evaluate the effectiveness of offering training and awareness programs for family members and educators. Offering short workshops to provide information about CSE may positively impact access to effective instruction for youth with IDDs and ASDs. In a recent study, results showed that most participants (educators/parents of youth with IDDs and ASDs) in a CSE workshop did provide sexuality education to their students/children following workshop attendance (Eyres et al. 2016).

PEOPLE WITH IDDS AND ASDS AND SEXUAL OFFENSES

Without a meaningful sex education, people with IDDs and ASDs are more likely to be the victim of sexual abuse (Swango-Wilson 2008) and are more likely to commit sexual abuse (Davis 2009). Swango-Wilson (2011) states people with IDDs and ASDs are four times more likely to be victims of sex crimes than people without IDDs. According to Swango-Wilson (2008), 39–60 percent of females and 16–30 percent of males with IDDs experience sexual abuse by age eighteen.

One of the reasons for the high incidence of sexual abuse for people with IDDs and ASDs is the fact they may not recognize abuse has occurred. Communication barriers may also contribute to the increase in sexual abuse since people with IDDs and ASDs may not be able to describe their experiences. The proximity of abusers also contributes to the high rate of sexual abuse. Females with IDD are most likely to be abused by caregivers (Swango-Wilson 2011).

Males who are abused often become aggressive in sexual encounters (Swango-Wilson 2011) and may perpetuate the cycle of physical abuse. According to Davis (2009), 10–15 percent of sexual offences are committed by people with IDD and ASD. Fifty percent of incarcerated people with IDDs and ASDs have committed sexual offences, and 34 percent of people with IDDs and ASDs in the community have committed sexual offences. The most common offences committed by people with IDDs and ASDs include inappropriate sexual behavior in public (62 percent), sexual behavior and simulation involving others (43 percent), sexual activity with minors (43 percent), and assaultive/nonconsensual activity not involving minors (35 percent).

There are a number of reasons for the sexual offences committed by people with IDDs and ASDs. According to Davis (2009), those reasons include lack of information, lack of social skills and training, a history of sexual or physical abuse, exposure to violence and pornography, socioeconomic factors, pervasive restriction, limited or no sexual partners, difficulty projecting consequences, and difficulty recognizing and expressing emotions. The fact significant others may deny that inappropriate behavior is happening is another reason such behavior may continue to occur.

EVIDENCE-INFORMED AND DATA-DRIVEN THEORY

Schaafsma, Stoffelen, Kok, and Curfs (2013) conducted a study of five sexuality education programs. They concluded none of the programs were theory- or evidence-based and that none of the programs had specific outcomes, a theoretical basis, or a systematic evaluation. Additionally, neither people with IDDs and ASDs nor their caregivers were involved in the development process of the programs. Schaafsma et al. (2013) determined none of the programs in the study would be effective.

Based on the results of their study, Schaafsma et al. (2013) made several recommendations. Successful sexuality education programs for people with IDDs and ASDs should include proper needs assessment in order to provide people with IDDs and ASDs with the information they require. They should focus on people with IDDs and ASDs and involve people with IDDs and ASDs in designing the programs. Finally, all programs should have measurable outcomes to conduct proper evaluations.

Educators/families should consider the following when selecting curricula/resources: (1) consider chronological age and developmental level; (2) utilize lessons from a variety of programs as needed per student; (3) use curricula as a guide and use evidence-based instructional strategies to deliver content; (4) build in opportunities for generalization of content skills learned (Blanchett and Wolfe 2002). Additionally, the Future of Sex Education

Chapter 5

Initiative (2012) offers a list of characteristics of effective sexuality education (figure 5.3).

Evaluating sexuality education curricula and/or programs under consideration is a helpful way of identifying whether it will meet the educational needs of students with IDD and/or ASD. A useful evaluation tool adapted from SIECUS is available in the book *Autism Spectrum Disorders*

CHARACTERISTICS OF EFFECTIVE SEXUALITY EDUCATION

Focuses on specific behavioral outcomes.

Addresses individual values and group norms that support health-enhancing behaviors.

Focuses on increasing personal perceptions of risk and harmfulness of engaging in specific health risk behaviors, as well as reinforcing protective factors.

Addresses social pressures and influences.

Builds personal and social competence.

Provides functional knowledge that is basic, accurate and directly contributes to health- promoting decisions and behaviors.

Uses strategies designed to personalize information and engage students.

Provides age-and developmentally-appropriate information, learning strategies, teaching methods and materials.

Incorporates learning strategies, teaching methods and materials that are culturally inclusive.

Provides adequate time for instruction and learning.

Provides opportunities to reinforce skills and positive health behaviors.

Provides opportunities to make connections with other influential persons.

Includes teacher information and plan for professional development and training to enhance effectiveness of instruction and student learning.

Figure 5.3 Characteristics of Effective Sexuality Education.
Future of Sex Education Initiative—Advocates for Youth, Answer, and the Sexuality Information and Education Council of the United States—National Sexuality Education Standards: Core Content and Skills, K–12, 2012, www.futureofsexed.org.

in Adolescents and Adults: Evidence Based and Promising Interventions, Chapter 9 Sexuality and Relationship for Individuals with Autism Spectrum Disorder (Travers and Whitbey 2015).

Sexuality Education Instruction: Tips and Suggestions

Specific instructional strategies for teaching sexuality education components mirror the same effective instructional strategies that work when students are taught other content (reading, math, science, etc.). The difference is not only the instructional strategies but also the content. Evidence-based practices such as task analysis, video modeling, visual supports, community-based generalization of skills learned at school, and prompting as needed are also effective when implementing sexuality education.

Basic accommodations assist in both content comprehension and retention. These can include *pacing of instruction* and *modified reading levels*. *Visuals* and *environmental supports* should be tailored to the individual students. Terms and materials should be *simple* and *concrete* and presented in *short time periods with small steps*, with *consistent repetition* and *opportunities to generalize*.

Studies of abstinence-only programs tend to be inconclusive or show them to be ineffective. Providing CSE does not lead to early or risky sexual activity (Breuner and Mattson 2016).

Helpful information/tips for families and educators when teaching sexuality education include the following:

- Keep it positive! (Especially if you disagree. *How you respond* is as important as what you say.)
- Discover the students' personal style in clothing and appearance.
- Do not "talk down" or imply incompetence.
- Allow for role-play and practice!
- Make room for individuality.
- Use correct terminology.
- Keep your sense of humor!

Remember if sexuality is being presented as negative or unnatural, the student may have trouble participating in society appropriately. Seek professional counseling help should the need arise (Baxley and Zendall 2011). It is important for students to know the correct names for body parts. Speaking or pointing to the correct body parts will better help the authorities (Baxley and Zendall 2011) should assistance be required.

COMPREHENSIVE TRANSITION PLANNING

The *transition planning process* focuses on educating students in terms of preparing for postschool life; it is comprehensive; requires support from home, school, and the community; and emphasizes autonomy (Lotstein et al. 2009). Federally mandated at age sixteen, transition planning must prepare adolescents and young adults with disabilities to utilize independent self-management skills to the best of their abilities as adults. Yet few transition programs for adolescents with IDDs or ASDs include information on reproductive or sexual health:

> For example, in a study, 34% of young adult women, 16 to 23 years, with type I diabetes stated they *knew "nothing" or were misinformed about diabetes and pregnancy*; 65% said they *knew nothing about preconception counseling*; and 63% said they *knew nothing about diabetes and birth control*. (Charron-Prochownik et al. 2006)

In another study, approximately 33 percent of adolescents had *annual physical exams without any mention of sexuality or sexual health*. Physicians and adolescents indicated *if there were discussions about reproductive health and sexuality, the conversations were brief* (Alexander et al. 2014). In another study, only 3 percent of adolescents *independently introduced topics of sexual behavior, STIs,* or *birth control with practitioners* (Merzel et al. 2004).

Oftentimes, transition practitioners do not recognize that their adolescents' developmental needs shifted during puberty (Sucato and Murray 2005). They may also assume the adolescent's sexual health is being addressed by outside providers. Most adolescents do not feel comfortable initiating conversations about sex with any kind of provider however, so it is imperative all members of the transition process work together to determine who will help adolescents and young adults with IDDs and ASDs manage their sexual health through adulthood.

Perhaps medical personnel are the logical choice to facilitate this kind of care, but one cannot assume that this concept is being "taken care of" by an outside provider. A survey of primary care physicians involved in transition programming reported that despite reproductive and sexual health being one of the most important issues for adolescents, many did not feel ready to educate their patients (Scal 2002). Without formal practices for sexual health education during the transition process, communication breakdowns can develop between providers and adolescents with IDDs and ASDs—ultimately limiting future outcomes for these students (Knapp et al. 2012).

See chapter 11 for a chart to get started on incorporating sexual health in the transition planning process.

EXAMPLES OF CURRICULA

Despite the results of Schaafsma et al. (2013), there are a number of sex education programs available attempting to meet the specific needs of people with IDDs and ASDs. A potentially useful instrument is the Socio-Sexual Knowledge and Attitudes Assessment Tool—Revised (SSKAAT-R; http://www.stoeltingco.com). This instrument, available through the Stoelting Company, is designed to measure "knowledge and attitudes of developmentally delayed and general populations, with emphasis on the setting of appropriate boundaries and behaviors."

Planned Parenthood has continued to provide resources for people with IDDs and ASDs. They utilize curricula from the Sexuality and Developmental Disabilities Workshops (http://disabilityworkshops.com/). In particular, the Sexuality Education for People with Developmental Disabilities Curriculum contains information on relationships and healthy sexual activities as well as the physical aspects of sexuality.

The Florida Developmental Disabilities Council has a downloadable sex education curriculum available on its website (www.albany.edu/aging/IDD/docs.htm). The curriculum includes units for various grade levels. The topics include Alike or Different (K-5), Changes in Your Body (4–8), Becoming an Adult (9–12), Beginning Social Skills (K-8), Advanced Social Skills (6–12), Dating, and Sexual and Physical Abuse. A copy of the caregiver version of the curriculum is included in the resources section of this module.

The Attainment Company (www.attainmentcompany.com) has produced a sex education curriculum for people with IDDs and ASDs called Learn About Life (LAL). The LAL curriculum is described as an illustrated sex education and social skills program for young adults with limited or no reading ability. The curriculum contains illustrations of topics to help individuals understand complicated facts of life.

The pictures are described as "tastefully but clearly illustrated" (www.attainmentcompany.com) and contain stickers to cover the illustration if it is deemed necessary to edit them. The LAL curriculum has six chapters: Your Body-My Body, Being a Woman, Being a Man, Having a Baby, Be Safe, and Relationships. Each chapter is divided into eight lessons. Each lesson contains objectives and teaching suggestions.

The Circles Curriculum (www.stanfield.com) consists of a video-modeling curriculum about social and relationship boundaries and relationship-specific social skills. The curriculum uses a simple multilayer circle diagram to demonstrate different relationship levels people with IDDs and ASDs encounter in their daily lives.

The curriculum is a concrete representation of different levels of interaction. One method of using the Circles Curriculum is to have people with IDDs and ASDs role-play levels of intimacy on color-coded floor mat. Similarly, people with IDDs and ASDs can create individualized posters representing the levels of intimacy in their own lives by writing names or attaching photograph of people in their lives onto a color-coded poster. The colors associated with each level of intimacy include purple: private; blue: family; green: friendship; yellow: acquaintances; orange: community helpers; red: strangers.

Safety Awareness for Empowerment (SAFE) is a curriculum developed by the Waisman Center at the University of Wisconsin—Madison. The eight-module curriculum teaches self-care and community safety, including safe relationships, avoiding victimization, and sexuality.

The Boy's Guide to Growing Up: Choices and Changes during Puberty (Couwenhoven 2012a) and *The Girls' Guide to Growing Up: Choices and Changes in the Tween Years* (Couwenhoven 2012b) are written on a third-grade reading level. The guides include activities to help tweens/teens learn about growing up.

The Healthy Bodies Toolkit for Girls and The Healthy Bodies Toolkit for Boys are developed by Vanderbilt University's Leadership Education in Neurodevelopmental Disabilities Consortium. The Toolkits are written for parents but can also be used by schools. Appendices in the Toolkits include storyboards and visuals.

The FLASH curriculum was developed by Public Health Seattle, King County. The curriculum includes an online comprehensive sexuality education curriculum with lesson plans, teacher guides, and trusted adult letters. It is aligned to both the CDC's National Health Education Standards for Sexual Health and the National Sexuality Education Standards.

Most of the sexuality education curricula presented so far stop short of providing information about the pleasurable aspects of sexuality and creating sexually healthy relationships. There are resources available to provide explicit instruction, as needed, for people with IDDs and ASDs. It has been recommended that curricula for people with IDDs and ASDs be individualized (AAIDD, 2008), be theory- or evidence-based, include proper needs assessment, and have measurable outcomes to conduct proper evaluations (Schaafsma et al. 2013).

The Diverse City Press (http://diverse-city.com) is a small publishing company of educational materials for people with IDDs and ASDs and caregivers. The publisher is linked to the disability rights movement and organizations and individuals promoting rights for people with IDDs and ASDs to take control of their lives. The Diverse City Press provides books and DVDs about sexuality. Their material is explicit and covers sensitive topics such as masturbation.

Sexuality and Relationship Education (SRE) (Hartman 2014) is a guide for children and adolescents with autism spectrum disorder, although the information presented is applicable to other people with IDDs and ASDs. SRE is research-based and grounded in applied behavior analysis. The book covers key sex education topics, including issues of gender, public and private behavior, puberty, hygiene, emotions, and the mechanics of sexual expression.

Hartman (2014) recommends beginning with a functional behavior assessment of the people with IDDs and ASDs, followed by the development of an individual behavior plan. The book provides task analyses of many hygiene and sexual situations. Additionally, the book provides social stories about relationships, hygiene, and sexual expression. There are reproducible forms and resources provided so that caregivers or teachers can individualize the education of an individual with IDD and ASD.

SRE is divided into four sections: (a) Understanding: supporting individuals in understanding issues involved in a best practice SRE program; (b) Preventing: concepts that should be included to prevent future issues; (c) Supporting: supporting individuals in developing healthy sexuality and intimate relationships; and (d) Responding: intervention tactics for responding to inappropriate sexualized behaviors

SRE planning should be embedded into a wider social skills program. SRE goals can be added to a person with IDD or ASD's Individual Education Program (IEP). The appendices of the book contain forms that can be used when planning, including checklists for the child and the organization conducting SRE, a functional behavior assessment, and an individual behavior plan. The appendices also contain illustrations about relationships, hygiene, and sexual expression, which may be used to create task analyses or social stories. Some of the illustrations are graphic or may depict sensitive topics. SRE recommends being sensitive to individuals' cultural, religious, and family values when selecting materials for use in lessons.

CONCLUSION

Sexuality education curricula specifically designed for students with IDDs and ASDs do exist; however, selection and implementation must be guided by individual student educational needs. Even the most effective curriculum must be modified to meet individual student needs/context. This will better prepare a person with IDD and ASD for living safely in the community.

INTERNET RESOURCES

1. Attainment Company: attainmentcompany.com/learn-about-life
2. Circles Curriculum: www.stanfield.com
3. Diverse City Press: diverse-city.com
4. Florida Developmental Disabilities Council, Inc.: (http://ceacw.org/docs/parentworkbook.pdf)
5. Planned Parenthood: plannedparenthood.org/planned-parenthood-northern-new-england/local-education-training/development-disabilites-sexuality
6. Socio-Sexual Knowledge and Attitudes Assessment Tool—Revised: stoeltingco.com

REFERENCES

AAIDD. (2008). Sexuality: Joint position statement of AAIDD and the Arc [Web page]. http://aaidd.org/news-policy/policy/position-statements/sexuality#. U2O5JFdhvzo.

Alexander S., Fortenberry J., Pollak K., Bravender, T., Davis, J., Ostbye, T., et al. (2014). Sexuality talk during adolescent health maintenance visits. *JAMA Pediatrics*, 168: 163–69.

Aunos, M., and Feldman, M. (2002). Attitudes towards sexuality, sterilization and parenting rights of persons with intellectual disabilities. *Journal of Applied Research on Intellectual Disabilities*, 15: 285–96.

Barnard-Brak, L., Schmidt, M., Chesnut, S., Wei, T., and Richman, D. (2014). Predictors of access to sex education for children with intellectual disabilities in public schools. *Intellectual and Developmental Disabilities*, 52: 85–97. doi:10.1352/1934–9556–52.2.85.

Barr, E. M., Goldfarb, E. S., Russell, S., Seabert, D., Wallen, M., and Wilson, K. L. (2014). Improving sexuality education: The development of teacher-preparation standards. *Journal of School Health*, 84: 396–415. DOI:10.1111/josh.12156.

Baxley, D., and Zendall, A. (2011). *Sexuality across the lifespan for children and adolescents with developmental disabilities*. Tallahasse, FL: Florida Developmental Disabilities Council, Inc.

Blanchett, W. J., and Wolfe, P. S. (2002). A review of sexuality education curricula: meeting the needs of individuals with moderate to severe intellectual disabilities. *Research and Practice for Persons with Severe Disabilities*, 27: 43–57.

Breuner, C. C., and Mattson G. (2016). Sexuality education for children and adolescents. *Pediatrics*, 138(2): e20161348. DOI: 10.1542/peds.2016–1348.

Charron-Prochownik D., Sereika S. M., Wang S. L., Hannan, M., Fischi, A., Stewart, S., and Dean-McElhinny, T. (2006). Reproductive health and preconception counseling awareness in adolescents with diabetes: What they don't know can hurt them. *Diabetes Education*, 32: 235–42.

Couwenhoven, T. C. (2012a). *The boy's guide to growing up: Choices and changes during puberty*. Bethesda, MD: Woodbine.

Couwenhoven, T. C. (2012b). *The girl's guide to growing up: Choices and changes in the tween years*. Bethesda, MD: Woodbine.

Davis, L. A. (2009). People with intellectual disabilities and sexual offenses http://www.thearc.org/page.aspx?pid=2456.

Elster, A., and Waltham, M. A. (2013). Guidelines for adolescent preventive services. Retrieved November 3, 2017. http://www.uptodate.com/contents/guidelines-for-adolescent-preventive-services.

Eyres, R., Williamson, R. L., Hunter, W., and Casey, L. (2016). Providing comprehensive sexuality education to students with intellectual and developmental disabilities: Preparing the trainer. *Division on Autism and Developmental Disabilities Online Journal*, 3(1): 160–71.

Future of Sex Education Initiative. (2012). National sexuality education standards: Core content and skills, K–12 [A special publication of the *Journal of School Health*]. http://www.futureofsexeducation.org/documents/josh-fose-standards-web.pdf.

Gougeon, N. A. (2009). Sexuality education for students with intellectual disabilities, a critical pedagogical approach: outing the ignored curriculum. *Sex Education*, 3: 177–291. DOI:10.1080/14681810903059094.

Hartman, D. (2014). *Sexuality and relationship education for children and adolescents with autism spectrum disorder*. London, England: Jessica Kingsley Publishers.

Howard-Barr, E., Rienzo, B. A., Pigg, R. M., and James, D. (2005). Teacher beliefs, professional preparation, and practices regarding exceptional students and sexuality education. *Journal of School Health*, 75: 99–104.

Knapp, C. A., Quinn, G. P., Rapalo, D., and Woodworth, L. (2012). Patient provider communication and reproductive health. In G. P. Quinn and S. T. Vadaparampil (Eds.), *Reproductive health and cancer in adolescents and young adults* (Vol. 732, 175–85). New York: Springer.

Lotstein, D. S., Ghandour, R., Cash, A., McGuire, E., Strickland, B., and Newacheck, P. (2009). Planning for health care transitions: Results from the 2005–2006 national survey of children with special health care needs. *Pediatrics*, 123: e145–52.

Merzel, C. R., VanDevanter, N. L., Middlestadt, S., Bleakley, A., Ledksy, R., and Messeri, P. (2004). Attitudinal and contextual factors associated with discussion of sexual issues during adolescent health visits. *Journal of Adolescent Health*, 35: 108–15.

Scal, P. (2002). Transition for youth with chronic conditions: Primary care physicians' approaches. *Pediatrics*, 110(6.2): 1315–21.

Schaafsma, D., Stoffelen, J. M. T., Kok, G., and Curfs, L. M. G. (2013). Exploring the development of existing sex education programmes for people with intellectual disabilities: An intervention mapping approach. *Journal of Applied Research in Intellectual Disabilities*, 26: 157–66. DOI:10.1111/jar.12017.

Sexuality Information and Education Council of the United States (SIECUS). (2004). *Guidelines for comprehensive sexuality education* (3rd ed.). Retrieved November 3, 2017. www.siecus.org.

Shtarkshall, R. A., Santelli, J. S., and Hirsch, J. S. (2007). Sex education and sexual socialization: Roles for educators and parents. *Perspectives on Sexual and Reproductive Health*, 39(2): 116–19.

Sucato, G., and Murray, P. (2005). Gynecologic health care for the adolescent solid organ transplant recipient. *Pediatric Transplantation*, 9: 346–56.

Swango-Wilson, A. (2008, June). Caregiver perception of sexuality behaviors of individuals with intellectual disabilities. *Sexuality and Disability*, 26(2): 75–81.

Swango-Wilson, A. (2011). Meaningful sex education programs for individuals with intellectual/developmental disabilities. *Sexuality and Disability*, 29: 113–18. DOI:10.1007/s11195-010-9168-2.

Travers, J., and Whitbey, P. (2015). Sexuality and relationships for individuals with autism spectrum disorders. In M. Tincani and A. Bondy, *Autism spectrum disorders in adolescents and adults: Evidence-based and promising interventions* (182–207). New York: Guilford.

United Nations Educational, Scientific and Cultural Organization (UNESCO). (2015). *Emerging evidence, lessons and practice in comprehensive sexuality education: A global review*. https://www.unfpa.org/sites/default/files/pub-pdf/CSE_Global_Review_2015.pdf.

Chapter 6

No One Can Escape Puberty: Physical and Cognitive Development

THE STORY OF TIA IN THE BATH

During bath playtime, Tia, a five-year-old girl with Down syndrome, is playfully squirting water. Her mother teaches Tia how to submerge the tip of the baster into the water while squeezing the bulb and then slowly releasing the bulb to fill the baster tube with water. Tia enjoys squirting the stream of water into the tub. She stands up and places the baster in front of her vagina and says, "My brother pees like this. He peed outside." Tia's mother asked if she peed outside too. Tia replied, "I sit down to pee. One day, I'm going to push his penis back inside him, so he can sit down to pee too."

Summary

All human beings are sexual beings and experience a complex process of sexual development guided by the nervous and endocrine systems. For individuals with intellectual or developmental disabilities (IDDs) and autism spectrum disorders (ASDs), physical sexual development follows a typical neurophysiological progression. This chapter provides an overview of the neurophysiological and neurocognitive aspects of healthy sexual development. Similarities and differences of the components of sexual development between individuals who are neurotypical and those who have an intellectual or developmental disability are identified.

Readers will develop an understanding of the following:

- Sexuality's four aspects: physical, emotional, social, and cultural.
- Neurophysiological sexual development's association with physical aspects of sexuality, and its division into an organization phase during prenatal development and activation phase during puberty.

- Neurophysiological sexual development and how it prepares the human body for the process of procreation.
- Neurocognitive sexual development that involves connections between the brain stem, limbic system, and cerebral cortex and develops continuously across the lifespan.
- Neurocognitive sexual development influences and is influenced by the emotional, social, and cultural aspects of sexuality.
- Individuals with and without IDDs experiences of the same process of neurophysiological sexual development, and many of the same processes of neurocognitive sexual development regulated at the level of brain stem, limbic, and endocrine system.
- Involvement of cerebral cortical regions of the brain, related to neurocortical sexual development, is where individuals with IDDs need developmentally appropriate, specialized, and individualized sexual education support.
- Individuals with IDDs are sexual beings who experience sexual attraction and sexual arousal, and should be supported in understanding how to engage in healthy, appropriate, and responsible sexual behaviors.

Across every developmental stage, humans are sexual beings. As sexual beings, human sexual development manifests anatomically, physiologically, psychologically, and cognitively. Sexual development consists of four interrelated components including emotional, social, cultural, and physical development. The four components of sexual development influence three aspects of sexuality, including sexual attraction, sexual arousal, and sexual behavior. Sexual development intersects with each of the four components and guides an individual's developmental sexuality (National Child Traumatic Stress Network 2009; The Society of Obstetricians and Gynecologists of Canada 2012).

The four components of sexual development are guided by neurophysiological and neurocognitive sexual development. From embryological stages through puberty, neurophysiological sexual development guides anatomical and physiological components of physical sexual development. Neurophysiological sexual development guides prenatal development of primary sex characteristics and the secondary sex characteristics that develop during puberty. Neurocognitive sexual development influences the emotional, social, and cultural aspects of sexual development across the lifespan.

NEUROPHYSIOLOGICAL ASPECTS
OF PHYSICAL SEXUAL DEVELOPMENT

There are two fundamental stages associated with development of the biological sex determination between males and females. These two stages define organizational differences and activation differences. Organizational differences are sex differences that occur during prenatal development, while activation effects occur during adolescence.

The anatomical differences that determine the biological sex assigned at birth are referred to as primary sex characteristics. These characteristics include both differences in internal and external organs of the reproductive system, which are unique to either males or females. These anatomical differences between the male and female reproductive organs result from a system of ducts and differing hormonal functions. The hormonal differences affect internal organ systems, which are hormonally activated to differentiate into characteristically male or female organs.

At the time of fertilization of an ova by a sperm, the genetic predispositions of male or female is determined by the haploid chromosome on the sperm, which carries either an X or Y chromosome. However, during the first three to four weeks of fetal development, the fetus is considered to be undifferentiated.

During this undifferentiated stage, the fetus has the potential to become either a male or a female. Differentiation begins with a specialized organ called the gonads. The gonads are referred to as bipotential structures during this undifferentiated stage of fetal development (Sadler 2015). By the tenth week of gestation, bipotential gonads develop into testes in males or ovaries in females.

Prenatal sexual development of primary sex characteristics can also be subject to a wide range of variability According to Roen and Pasterski (2014), approximately 2 percent of live births are identified as having a disorder of sex development (DSD), also referred to as intersex (Beh and Milton 2014). In the absence of anti-Müllerian hormone, female reproductive organs will develop, regardless of the sex-determining chromosomes.

Examples of DSD in the external genitalia include a urethral opening that appears in a place other than the tip of the penis or a clitoris that appears visibly larger than the norm, resembling a penis (Beh and Milton 2014; Roen and Pasterski 2014). However, many forms of DSD are not identified until adolescence or later in life. The anatomical variation impacts the internal organs, which is not apparent from visual observation of the external anatomical structures.

When an infant is born, the primary sex characteristics of the reproductive organs are organizationally prepared for reproduction. The female ovaries contain their full complement of ova, and the testes are organizationally prepared for spermatogenesis. As a result of this organizational development, infants experience physiological aspects of sexual arousal (DeLamater and Friedrich 2002). Erection of the male infant's penis is common, and vaginal lubrication of the vagina has been reported in female infants within 24 hours after birth (Masters, Johnson, and Kolodny 1982).

Characteristic infantile behavior such as infants sucking their fingers or toes and soothing human interactions such as being cuddled, massaged, and rocked are described by DeLamater and Friedrich as sexual experiences that may establish preferences for various means of stimulation that may persist throughout life.

The neurophysiological aspect of physical sexual development prepares female and male human beings for the biological process of procreation of the species. When the organizational phase of physical sexual development is complete at birth and the activational phase begins in early adolescence, the human body is physically prepared for the biological process of sexual reproduction. Children and adolescents with IDDs experience typical organizational and activational phases of the physical component of sexual development along the same developmental trajectory as their neurotypical peers.

NEUROCOGNITIVE OF SOCIAL, EMOTIONAL, AND CULTURAL SEXUAL DEVELOPMENT

Social, emotional, and cultural components of sexual development are associated with neurocognitive brain development. These components of neurocognitive sexual development involve integrated connections between the brain stem, limbic system, and the cerebral cortex.

The aspects of sexuality that are controlled by neurocognitive sexual development include sexual attraction, sexual arousal, and sexual behavior. Neurocognitive connections between various brain regions influence and coordinate sexual attraction, sexual arousal, and sexual behavior. The brain stem controls basic life functions that are autonomically regulated, meaning without conscious control. Examples of autonomic regulation include breathing, attention, and reflexive motor responses.

A long, narrow network of neurons known as the reticular formation runs through the brain stem. The reticular formation is responsible for filtering out some of the stimuli that comes into the brain from the spinal cord and relaying the remainder of the signals to other areas of the brain. The reticular formation plays important roles in walking, eating, sexual activity, and sleeping.

With respect to sexual activity, the reticular formation connects to parts of the limbic system, which regulates emotions and behaviors related to emotions. This filtering of sensory information by the reticular formation, with respect to sexual attraction, brings attention to sensory stimulation that triggers physical and romantic attractions of an individual toward a potential sexual partner.

According to the Society of Obstetricians and Gynaecologists of Canada (2017), sexual attraction is uniquely defined by each individual, and neurologically controlled by interactions between the reticular formation and the limbic areas of the brain. Uniquely defined sexual attraction is based on multiple factors: physical appearance, an individual's voice tone or smell, the clothing an individual wears, what culture they are from, and their personality, charm, and politeness.

The complexities of what constitutes sexual attraction are endless and contribute to the diversity of human sexuality. Through continual neurocognitive sexual development, individuals begin to recognize and define what they consider sexually attractive, and these attractions can change over time. Sexual orientation categorizes different types of sexual attraction based on a person's assigned biological sex.

Sexual arousal is influenced by sexually attractive sensory stimuli. Sexual arousal usually begins with the neurocognitive response to a thought or image, having a feeling of closeness or affection toward a partner or by the touch of a partner. The process of arousal is physiologically initiated by sending hormonal signals, particularly to the ovaries and testes to release estrogen in females or testosterone in males.

Physiological responses to sexual arousal include an erection for males. Swelling of the nipples, vulva, and clitoris and vaginal lubrication occur when females are sexually aroused (The Society of Obstetricians and Gynaecologists of Canada 2017).

The hypothalamus is part of the limbic system. In addition to triggering the release of hormones from the pituitary gland, the hypothalamus also interacts with other parts of the limbic system to regulate autonomic feelings like hunger, thirst, and sexual arousal. The hypothalamus is commonly referred to as the brain's pleasure center, because the hypothalamus responds to the satisfaction of these basic human needs by creating a feeling of pleasurable satisfaction (Swenson 2006).

Sensory input that is perceived as sexually attractive to an individual triggers the limbic system to physiologically prepare for sexual arousal. The hypothalamic connections relay this information through the limbic and endocrine systems subconsciously.

The physiological effects of sexual arousal, such as vaginal lubrication or penile erection, are limbic responses of sexual arousal. Arousal physiologically prepares the body for pleasurable sexual behavior. Sexual arousal and orgasms are regulated by the limbic system and can occur without conscious control. It is typical, especially during adolescence, to have dreams with sexually arousing images or scenarios, which can cause the same physiological responses of sexual arousal and ejaculation, commonly referred to as wet dreams.

The cerebral cortex, particularly the frontal lobe, regulates cognitive thought processes, and integrates new information learned from new knowledge and experiences. Children begin to learn social and cultural expectations and norms related to sexuality through observation and experiences. The way adults respond to sexualized behaviors, culture expectations of gender roles, clothing that is considered age-appropriate, family values, media influence, and peer interactions contribute to the development of an individual's neurocognitive sexual development. The sexual development is a complex process that continually evolves throughout the lifespan (Kar, Choudhury, and Singh 2015).

The cerebral cortex plays an important role in neurocognitive sexual development. Cognitive and psychological development control how an individual inhibits or pursues sexual behaviors that arise from sexual attractions and sexual arousal. Understanding the cognitive and psychological functions of neurocognitive sexual development is important for parents, educators, and caregivers to support neurocognitive sexual development.

Brain anatomy is divided into grey matter and white matter. As the brain functionally develops, the presence of white matter increases. White matter represents the myelination of the axons of neurons. The myelinated axons form pathways between various brain regions. The white matter between the cerebral cortex and limbic system is referred to as corticolimbic pathways. A longitudinal study of the development of white matter in children between the ages of eight and twenty demonstrated that late maturation of corticolimbic connections supports the socioemotional sexual immaturity of typical childhood and early adolescence (Simmonds et al. 2014).

Cerebral cortical neurocognitive sexual development is necessary for understanding the connections between matters such as personal hygiene, appropriate and inappropriate forms of physical contact, and public versus private aspects of sexual behavior. For individuals with neurotypical cognitive development, many of the social and cultural aspects of neurocognitive sexual development are learned through observation.

However, comprehensive sexual education is important for higher order critical thinking related to the complexity of sexuality (Kar, Choudhury, and Singh 2015). Individuals with an intellectual or developmental disability have difficulty with understanding social and cultural norms without explicit, specialized, and individualized instruction.

Explicit, developmentally appropriate comprehensive sexuality education is as important for individuals with IDD and ASD as it is for children who are neurotypical. They have sexual attractions, experience sexual arousal, and need to understand appropriate public and private sexual behaviors. Explicit instruction regarding sexual attraction, sexual arousal, and sexual behavior is necessary to understand appropriate social interactions with a person to whom they may feel sexually attracted.

CONCLUSION

Sexual education for individuals with IDD and ASD should begin in early childhood. Children with intellectual disabilities, like neurotypical children, explore their bodies. Oftentimes, the discovery of the pleasurable sensation of fondling their genitals results in masturbation in public, or removing their clothing in the presence of other people.

Teaching young children that touching certain parts of their body is appropriate in private, but not in public or in the presence of other people is an example of developmentally appropriate sexual education. For individuals with IDD and ASD, understanding these social and cultural aspects of appropriate sexual behavior requires consistent, explicit direct instruction.

As children approach puberty, specialized instruction is needed for individuals with IDD and ASD to understand the physical development of secondary sex characteristics that emerge during puberty. However, it is not uncommon for adolescents and adults with IDD and ASD to be treated as a perpetual child in a maturing body. Most aspects of sexual attraction, sexual arousal, and the desire for pleasurable sexual behaviors are equivalent to the pleasure-seeking hypothalamic functions associated with other autonomic sensations associated with basic human needs (Kar, Choudhury, and Singh 2015).

Comprehensive, inclusive sexual education is important for individuals with IDDs to understand the physical, emotional, social, and cultural aspects of sexual development. Parents, educators, and caregivers also need to be trained to understand the similarities and differences that promote healthy sexual development for individuals with IDDs and ASDs. Table 6.1 provides developmentally appropriate guidelines for supporting sexual development.

RESOURCES

Internet Resources

SexEd Library: sexedlibrary.org
- Sexuality Information and Education Council of the United States (SIECUS) provides the SexEd Library, which is a comprehensive online sex education resources on human sexuality. Resources in the SexEd Library include lesson plans, information and statistics, and professional development opportunities related to human sexuality.

Books/Articles and Other Resources

The *Sexuality and Safety with Tom and Ellie* a series by Kate E. Reynolds:
- *Things Ellie Likes*: A book about sexuality and masturbation for girls and young women with autism and related conditions.

Table 6.1 Developmentally Appropriate Guidelines for Supporting Sexual Development

	Neurophysiological sexual development	Neurocognitive sexual development
Preschool children (less than 4 years)	• Boys and girls have different body parts • Accurate names for body parts of boys and girls • Private parts are your body parts that are covered by a bathing suit or underwear • Babies grow inside mommies first • Simple answers to questions about the body and bodily functions	• The difference between "okay" touches (which are comforting, pleasant, and welcome) and "not okay" touches (which are intrusive, uncomfortable, unwanted, or painful) • Your body belongs to you • No one—child or adult—has the right to touch your private parts • It is okay to say "no" when adults ask you to touch their private parts, or for them to touch or kiss your private parts • Who to tell if people do "not okay" things to you or ask you to do "not okay" things to them
Young children (4–6 years)	• Boys' and girls' bodies change when they get older • Simple explanations of how babies grow in their mother's womb and about the birth process	• There are different types of hugs and kisses • You have the right to say no to anyone who tries to hug you, kiss you, or touch your private parts • Touching your own private parts can feel nice; it is okay in private and when you are alone
Older children/ preteens (ages 7–12)	• What to expect and how to handle changes of puberty (including menstruation and wet dreams) • Basics of reproduction, pregnancy, and childbirth • Risks of sexual activity (pregnancy and sexually transmitted diseases)	• There are different types of relationships (family, friendships, romantic relationships) • Hugs and kisses, even with family members, change as you get older • Understanding sexual attraction and arousal • How clothing and social interactions relate to attraction
Teens (13–18)	• Understanding the processes of sexual behaviors • Have a person who they are comfortable asking questions about sexual attraction, arousal, and behavior	• Social opportunities to explore potential romantic relationships • Opportunities to talk about and explore sexuality • Understanding how to seek consent and how to give consent
Young Adults (19–21)	• Ability to self-determine sexuality • Continued support for questions about sexual attraction, arousal, and behavior • Opportunities for privacy and intimacy	• Ability to explore and pursue romantic relationships • Inclusion in social and cultural aspects of sexuality, relationships, and family planning

- *Things Tom Likes*: A book about masturbation for boys and young men with autism and related conditions.
- *What's Happening to Ellie?* A book about puberty for girls and young women with autism and related conditions.
- *What's Happening to Tom?* A book about puberty for boys and young men with autism and related conditions.
- *Sexuality and Severe Autism A Practical Guide for Parents, Caregivers and Health Educators.*

Suggestions for How to Remain Current on This Topic

- Remain current on your state laws and policies related to sex education.
- Advocate for inclusive sex education in your school district or school site.
- Follow the organizations listed below on social media, and sign up for Kinsley Institute Newsletter to remain current on research related to human sexuality.
- Resources to help you stay current:

  – American Association of Sexuality Educators, Counselors, and Therapists; aasect.org
  – Kinsley Institute (Indiana University); kinsleyinstitute.org
  – Planned Parenthood; plannedparenthood.org
  – Society for the Scientific Study of Sexuality (SSSS); sexscience.org

REFERENCES

Beh, H.G., and Milton, D. (2014, Fall). Individuals with differences in sex development: Consult to Columbia Constitutional Court regarding sex and gender. *Wisconcin Journal of Law, Gender, & Society*, 29(3): 421–445.

DeLamater, J., and Friedrich, W. N. (2002). Human sexual development. *The Journal of Sex Research*, 39(1): 10–14. http://www.jstor.org/stable/3813417.

Kar, S. K., Choudhury, A., and Singh, A. P. (2015). Understanding normal development of adolescent sexuality: A bumpy ride. *Journal of Human Reproductive Sciences*, 8(2): 70–74. DOI: 10.4103/0974-1208.158594.

Masters, W. H., Johnson, V. E., and Koldny R. C. (1986). *Masters and Johnson on sex and human loving*. New York: Little Brown.

National Child Traumatic Stress Network. (2009). *Sexual development and behavior in children: Information for parents and caregivers*. Retrieved from the Alaska Department of Health and Social Services, Office of Children's Services: http://hss.state.ak.us/ocs/Publications/pdf/ sexualdevelop-children.pdf.

Roen, K., and Pasterski, V. (2014). Psychological research and intersex/DSD: Recent developments and future directions. *Psychology and Sexuality*, 5(1): 102–16. DOI: 10.1080/19419899.2013.831218.

Sadler, T. W. (2015). *Langman's medical embryology*, 13th ed. Philadelphia, PA: Wolters Kluwer.

Simmonds, D., Hallquist, M. N., Asoto, M., and Luna, B. (2014). Developmental stages and sex differences of white matter and behavioral development through adolescence: A longitudinal diffusion tensor imaging (DTI) study. *Neuroimage*, 92: 356–368. DOI: 10.1016/j.neuroimage.2013.12.044.

The Society of Obstetricians and Gynaecologists of Canada. (2017). *Sexuality and childhood development*. Retrieved November 3, 2017. http://www.sexualityandu. ca/ parents/sexuality-child-development.

Swenson, R. (2006). *Review of clinical and functional neuroscience*. Dartmouth, NH: Dartmouth Medical School.

Chapter 7

What Does It All Mean?: LGBTQ+

Sarah, a thirty-year-old woman with an autism spectrum disorder diagnosis, goes to her new doctor. Upon the initial health interview with the nurse practitioner, it is discovered that Sarah used to be called Steven. Sarah reports that despite her male body parts, she began to identify as female as young as the age of three. Her parents and educators blamed her diagnosis of autism for the "gender confusion" and would not allow Sarah to portray herself as female. Now Sarah lives on her own and is fully identifying as female. She still has male genitalia but would like to explore gender-reassignment surgery.

Further discussion reveals that Sarah is using the Internet to seek out sexual relationships. When asked about her sexual orientation, she insists she is heterosexual and goes on to explain that she is finding men on the Internet. Sarah described one occasion where she invited a man to her home, and he was physically abusive after discovering she had a penis.

Clearly, Sarah is dealing with a series of issues that may pose challenges to the health care provider. The health care provider must seek out ways to support not only Sarah's sexual behavior and health but also her gender identification. She no longer has a relationship with her parents and is unable to report any kind of support system.

How can the health care provider support Sarah's sexual health alongside her gender identity?

SUMMARY

Talking about one's gender identity and sexuality can be a particularly effective way of advocating for oneself, as it is such a personal subject (Azzopardi-Lane and Callus 2014). However, for these individuals, sexual and gender identity is often assumed and prescribed by others. Little opportunity is provided for individuals with IDDs and ASDs to understand and explore gender or sexual variance.

Similarly, because of developmental delays or cognitive impairment, parents and caregivers often attempt to protect individuals from sexual abuse or inappropriate sexual behavior with protective or avoidant behavior. This ultimately results in individuals with IDDs and ASDs lacking education and opportunities to use self-advocacy skills to explore and define their unique sexuality and gender. Consequently, individuals with IDDs and ASDs often have a sequestered sexuality.

This chapter reviews gender identity development and sexuality development in the context of a construct referred to as gender and sexuality diversity (GSD). By the end of this chapter, readers will be able to:

- define terminology that promotes meaningful understanding of gender and sexuality development from a non-binary perspective;
- identify nonbinary perspective of gender identity formation and sexuality development;
- distinguish how GSD affects individuals with IDD and ASD;
- identify strategies to promote inclusive GSD in school environments.

GENDER IDENTITY

GSD, an inclusive construct acknowledging the centrality of gender and sexuality in all human beings, is an essential and inherently diverse aspect of a person's identity (Bryan 2012). The development of a gender identity is a complex process involving both biological and psychological factors (Diamond 2006; Freeman and Knowles 2012).

Diamond (2006) described this integration of nature and nurture in the development of gender identity as biased interaction theory (BIT). BIT posits an infant is born with a determined evolutionary heritage, genetic inheritance, and uterine environmental influences yielding a propensity for expression of certain gender and sexuality patterns. Yet, the gender and sexuality preferences that are eventually expressed by the individual are influenced by upbringing and societal values.

The assigned biological sex refers to the anatomical and physiological characteristics that define males and females, while gender refers to society's constructed roles, expectations, behaviors, attitudes, and activities that it deems appropriate for men and women. As soon as the biological sex of a fetus is assigned either from a uterine ultrasonic examination during pregnancy or from observation of the neonate's external genitalia at birth, the tendency is for parents and others to begin to make gender-based decisions for their child.

For example, the parents select a name for their daughter or son, purchasing gendered clothing, furnishings, and decorations. Toys and gifts for the baby align to the societal assumptions of the preferences of either boys or girls.

Gender expectations also influence how infants are perceived soon after birth. Boys are perceived as strong and masculine, while girl infants tend to be perceived as fragile and dainty. These environmental influences on gender expectations influence the child's understanding of gender expectations. By the age of two, most children show awareness of their own gender, prefer gender-stereotyped toys, and tend to imitate culturally influenced gender behaviors of familiar activities (Bryan 2012).

The first self-awareness of gender may be an article of clothing that may feel too "boyish" or "girlish" to wear, while for others it may be noticing certain behaviors such as preferences for playing with trucks and cars rather than dolls or realizing the societal expectations that encourage boys to play with trucks and action figures. Gender is incorporated into all aspects of daily life from birth onward and can be socially uncomfortable if we are unsure of someone's gender or have issues coming to understand our own (Bedard, Hui, and Zucker 2010; Diamond 2016).

Gender Binary

Western cultural beliefs dictate there are only two biological sexes directly corresponding to two distinct genders. A person who is assigned the biological sex of girl is considered to have the gender of a female, and a biological assignment of boy equates to the male gender. This is referred to as the *gender binary* (Bryan 2015). The binary pairing of biological sex and gender is assumed to determine an individual's sexual attraction to the opposite sex-gender coupling.

Women are expected to have gender identification of females and are expected to be attracted to men. Similarly, men are expected to have gender identification of male and be attracted to women. These assumed binary correlations between sex, gender, and sexuality are referred to as *heteronormative assumptions*. Any variation that does not correlate to these binary couplings between biological sex, gender, and sexuality has historically been considered unnatural or pathological (Dragowski, Sharrón-del Rio, and Sandingorsky 2011).

According to the construct of GSD, most individuals identify with some combination of characteristics, personality traits, and preferences that society categorizes as masculine or feminine. Typically, when asked to identify one's gender, the binary choices of male or female are provided.

Byran (2015) reports a study of college students who were asked to identify their gender on a binary scale of male, female, or other. When given only these three choices, 98 percent selected either male or female. Only 2 percent defined their gender as "other" or nonconforming to the gender binary. When the same study participants were given a continuum scale with male at one end of the spectrum and female at the other end, 20 percent of participants defined their gender identity as falling somewhere in the middle, not fully female or male (Bryan 2015).

Some individuals feel strongly their assigned biological sex is incongruent with their gender identity (Richards and Barker 2015). When an individual chooses to live their life expressing the gender they identify with, rather than the gender typically coupled with their assigned sex, the individual may identify as *transgender*. *Transgender* is a nonmedical term that has been commonly used since the 1990s as a general term describing individuals whose gender identity (inner sense of gender) or gender expression (outward performance of gender) differs from the sex or gender to which they were assigned at birth (Drescher and Pula 2017).

Language and culture of the lesbian, gay, bisexual, and transgender (LGBTQ) community are continually evolving. As alternatives to the gender binary are explored, new terminology has emerged including gender expansive, gender fluid, gender variant, gender creativity, genderqueer, bigender, and agender, which are increasingly used to express the diversity of genders that do not conform to the traditional gender binary attribution (Drescher and Pula 2017; Freeman and Knowles 2012).

Gender Dysphoria

The fifth edition of the *Diagnostic and Statistical Manual of Mental Disorders* (*DSM-5*) introduced the term *gender dysphoria* (GD) as the medical term for transgender. GD replaced a previous diagnostic term *gender identity disorder* represented in previous editions of the *DSM*. The change in terminology reflects advocacy of the LGBT community's argument that being transgender is not a pathology or impairment, rather the diversity of gender and sexuality represents biodiversity represented in the natural variation that characterizes many human characteristics such as shoe size, hair color, facial features, and skin tone.

However, a medical term is needed for doctors to prescribe medical treatment such as hormone suppression therapy or, for some, gender reassignment surgery, which provides the option for transgender individuals to live in a body expressing the gender correlated to their identity. Therefore, GD reflects the personal conflict the individual experiences between their gender identity and assigned biological sex. Having GD is not the same as gender nonconformity and does not have any correlation to the individual's sexual orientation (Parekh 2016).

According to Drescher and Pula (2017), "Not all transgender people suffer from GD and that distinction is important to keep in mind. Gender dysphoria and/or coming out as transgender can occur at any age."

Sometimes, individuals who do not conform to the gender binary consider their gender to be something other than male or female. For example, the individual may have a preference for gender-neutral pronouns such as the singular *they/their/them* or "ze" (or "zie") and "hir" as opposed to *he/him/his* or *she/her/hers*. Other individuals may feel gender fluid, meaning their gender identity fluctuates between feeling more male at times and more female at other times. The flux could be a day-to-day fluctuation or a different gender expression during various stages of the individual's life.

Occasionally, very young children begin expressing their self-expression of being a different gender as soon as they develop gender awareness. Others may develop a growing awareness of being transgender later in their development. Parekh (2016) states cross-gender behaviors may start between ages two and four, the typical developmental stage when children begin showing gendered behaviors and interests. The personal acceptance of being transgender is also influenced by the type of opportunities the individual has to explore gender roles and to explore their personal gender expression.

Gender attribution is the perception others have of a person's gender identity, based on their gender expression. The research of Vries, Steensma, Cohen-Kettenis, VanderLaan, and Zucker (2016) shows children who had intense symptoms of distress, who were persistent, insistent, and consistent in their cross-gender statements and behaviors, and who use more declarative statements "I am a boy (or girl)" rather than "I want to be a boy (or girl)" were more likely to become transgender adults.

How Cognitive Impairments Affect Gender Development

Throughout childhood, predictable stages of play correspond to typical developmental stages. Gender development includes defining and understanding one's own gender identity, as well as increasing complexity of understanding gender attribution and gender expression.

Through pretend and imaginary play, children explore and learn about their environment, cultural and societal expectations, including gender roles (Bryan 2012; Kothlow and Chamberlain 2012). Typically, as children enter the developmental stage of pretend and imaginary play, they begin to show a preference for playing with same-gendered peers, who share similar interests.

Developmental stages, including stages of play behavior, are frequently delayed in children with IDDs and ASDs. Consequently, the exploration of gender roles may also be delayed until the child developmentally enters the stage of pretend play and imaginary play. However, awareness of gender identity and gender attribution, such as preferences for certain types of toys, characters, or clothing, can develop between the ages of two and four, similar to their neurotypical peers (Jahoda and Pownall 2014).

Individuals with IDDs and ASDs may also not intuitively learn about differences in gender roles, for example, developing learned social expectations of typical socially assigned gender roles of men and women, such as family structure (every child has one mother and one father); typical occupations for men and women; expected behaviors and capabilities of boys or girls, men or women; and so on.

For individuals with IDDs and ASDs, opportunities for exploration of gender expression can be limited. If a young girl with IDD or ASD says, "I'm a boy," this statement is often corrected, assuming that the child is just confused about gender terminology (Sherer et al. 2015). The child with IDD or ASD often has fewer opportunities to make decisions about what clothing to purchase or to wear. Parents and caregivers make these decisions based on gender attribution that correlates to the assigned biological sex.

SEXUAL IDENTITY AND ORIENTATION

Sexual attraction refers to the gender or genders a person is attracted to either physically or romantically and can occur independently of one another. A man might find a woman to be physically attractive but not be romantically attracted to her. Likewise, a woman may be romantically attracted to women but may find all forms of gender expression physically attractive.

Sexual orientation is the control of attractions, arousal, and behavior, and is demonstrated through emotional and physical attractions (Bryan 2015). Sexual arousal is the physical reaction to an attraction and leads to sexual behavior, the physical actions. Sexual behavior can be either with oneself (masturbation) or with a sexual partner. Neurologically, sexual arousal occurs without awareness or control, but higher-order neurological processes (executive functioning) control sexual behaviors. An example of this is obtaining consent from a sexual partner, ensuring privacy for sexual behavior, or generalizing skills and strategies for maintaining sexual maturity (Niles and Harkins Monaco 2017).

Similar to gender, sexuality is multifaceted and expansive and does not conform to a binary. New vocabulary is emerging to express the diversity of sexual orientations, beyond the binary of heterosexuality or homosexuality including concepts such as bisexuality or pansexuality.

Everyone has a sexual orientation; people who identify as heterosexual are attracted to individuals of the opposite sex, while those who identify as homosexual are attracted to individuals of the same sex. People who are *bisexual* are attracted to both sexes, and individuals who are attracted to all forms of gender expression identify as *pansexual*. It is possible to not be sexually aroused by any gender, which is referred to as *asexuality*, or perhaps an individual "questions" or expresses confusion about sexual orientation. Some people staunchly identify with a particular orientation, while others experience more fluidity (Planned Parenthood 2017).

How Cognitive Impairments Affect Sexual Development

Individuals with IDDs and ASDs are frequently overlooked as sexual beings despite having developed as an area of research and social policy, which in itself promotes the concept that individuals with IDDs and ASDs are sexual beings (Richards and Barker 2015). This population historically has experienced limitations with sexual maturity however, and many individuals with IDDs and ASDs cannot relate to cultural standards of gendered or sexual behavior (Planned Parenthood 2017).

Outside biases are hard for most people to recognize, as they have been unconsciously exposed prior to birth; students with IDDs and ASDs especially may not be aware. They most likely will not recognize how societal and psychosocial barriers interfere with individual development—personal or social, and this lack of understanding ultimately impacts their tolerance for others' gender or sexual identity and expression. This heteronormativity is powerful and impacts cultural norms, societal expectations, and relationships (Bryan 2012).

TEACHING STRATEGIES

If schools are to prioritize the development of the whole child—socially, emotionally, and academically—then challenging heteronormative assumptions should also be prioritized. Just as individuals who experience marginalization based on disability, race, ethnicity, religion, individuals are also marginalized based on heteronormative assumptions of gender identity or sexual diversity.

School environments have been described by Kothlow and Chamberlain (2012) as asexual, but the concept of gender and sexuality in schools has historically been hidden or largely ignored. The first step in supporting diverse sexual and gender identity and orientation in school is to teach using a comprehensive sexuality curriculum and establish inclusive cultures encompassing concepts in gender and sexuality.

People with IDDs and ASDs are often discouraged from exploring their sexuality, which means they are not safely and appropriately learning how to manage their personal sexuality. Educators can model and influence appropriate sexual practices by implementing the guidelines in table 7.1:

Table 7.1   Recommendations to Build Empathy and Promote Diversity

Encourage students to . . .	*By modeling or creating this*
Build empathy	• Create safe and welcoming classroom environments • Recognize and address heteronormative assumptions • Avoid unintentionally creating sexist or homophobic classroom environments
Promote inclusive diversity	• Incorporate tolerant curricula and literature • Emphasize examples that honor nontraditional gender roles • Foster understanding of gender nonconforming variations to the gender binary; use examples that range from male to female and heterosexual to homosexual • Create explicit expectations in the classroom that everyone deserves respect, especially considering elements of gender or sexual identity or expression • Address specific societal stereotypes that limit students, their sexual health, and their tolerance for others • Include biological, social, and legal factors of sexual and gender expression

(Luyckx, Vansteenkiste, Goossens, and Duriez, 2009; Niles and Harkins Monaco 2017)

INCLUSIVE AND SUPPORTIVE SCHOOL COMMUNITIES

When educators provide opportunities to establish and respect personal value systems collaboratively, the entire school community is capable of embracing GSD. Schools can shape and cultivate aspects of GSD by advertising elements of inclusive diversity on bulletin boards and announcements; through literature, library resources, and curriculum; and through general conversations and decorum.

Student clubs and activities can embrace tolerance through open discussions and acceptance of students who have flexible sexual or gender expression or identity; administrators can offer training opportunities for students, parents, and faculty and staff on gender identity and sexual orientation, and can identify community members (e.g., family members, friends, service providers, advocacy groups) who can help students navigate this process safely at the appropriate cognitive level (American Psychological Association 2017; Niles and Harkins Monaco 2017; Planned Parenthood 2017).

School policies prohibiting discrimination are common, but many do not emphasize sexual orientation, gender identity, or gender expression. It is important to work *with* students to establish these inclusive policies, but students typically inherit value systems and are expected to do as they are told. Rules are usually posted prior to the beginning of the school year, inadvertently supporting feelings of helplessness or a lack of control. This can be especially limiting for individuals who have IDDs and ASDs, who are often dependent on others to understand rights, responsibilities, or morals that support the school's values or mission.

Negative school cultures not only hamper students' academic achievements but also interfere with their emotional well-being. This is drastically increased for students who do not identify with the traditional gender binary:

- Around 75.1 percent of transgender students feel unsafe at school because of gender expression.
- Around 63.4 percent of transgender students reported avoiding bathrooms.
- Around 41 percent of transgender or gender non-conforming people have attempted suicide (*Gender Spectrum* 2016).

These experiences are all-encompassing beyond traditional classroom experiences. In fact, students' right to use bathrooms consistent with their gender identities is one that is specifically relevant in the current political climate.

Bathroom Laws

In May 2016, the U.S. Department of Education issued a formal statement to the nation's schools stating transgender students should be allowed to use the school bathrooms matching their gender identity, citing a federal law that protects students from gender discrimination. There were immediate responses to this. Thirteen states challenged these guidelines and the Department of Justice sued North Carolina over its "bathroom law," which prohibited municipal governments from passing laws that protect the rights of transgender people and mandated that people in government facilities use the bathrooms corresponding to their biological sex.

In February of 2017, however, the U.S. Department of Education under President Trump dropped the federal lawsuit filed against North Carolina and withdrew federal support for President Obama's ordinance, citing states' rights. State legislatures, including Virginia, New Hampshire, Colorado, Texas, North Carolina, Ohio, Wisconsin, and Pennsylvania, have since reviewed restroom bills.

The highest-profile restroom case to date is Virginia's G.G. v. Gloucester County School Board. Gavin Grimm, a high school senior in Virginia who is transgender, was previously allowed—with permission from his high school principal—to use the boys' bathroom at school. Enough parents complained, however, to warrant a school board ruling that students could only use bathrooms corresponding with their biological sex or a separate single-stall restroom.

In February 2017, the U.S. Supreme Court chose not to rule on the case, stating the U.S. Court of Appeals for the Fourth Circuit should be given another opportunity to hear Grimm's case. This case is currently pending (American Civil Liberties Union 2017).

CONCLUSION

If some people have the right to explore and understand personal gender and sexual identity, we must value *everyone's* rights for expression, identity, and personal sexual satisfaction—including those with IDDs and ASDs. These individuals have the right to explore personal gender identity and sexuality too, but understanding and navigating the complexities of gender and sexuality diversity can be challenging.

Full understanding of sexual diversity requires opportunities to experience and explore feelings of sexual attraction and sexual arousal, something that is often not an option for students with IDDs and ASDs. School communities can support the free expression of gender and sexual identity by establishing practices, utilizing resources, and creating opportunities for self-defined expressions of unique individuality.

RESOURCES

There are several organizations promoting awareness about sexuality and gender diversity:

- *The Ackerman Institute for the Family: The Gender and Family Project* has gender-inclusive resources; trainings; curricula for elementary, middle, and high school classrooms; and resources for families and caregivers. It also provides literature that explores more gender diversity across a variety of reading comprehension levels: ackerman.org/gfp/.
- *Planned Parenthood* is a nonprofit organization that delivers reproductive health care, sexuality education, and sexual orientation and gender identity resources: plannedparenthood.org/learn/teens/lgbtq/.

- The *Gender Spectrum* website offers trainings, books, multimedia resources, and additional conference opportunities that support gender-sensitive and gender-inclusive environments (https://www.genderspectrum.org/).

There are a variety of books that help support youth's sexual and gender exploration, but it is important to start this process as early as possible. The following picture books can assist young students navigate same-sex relationships:

- *King and King* by Linda de Haan and Stern Nijland. 2004. Gr. 2–5.
  A prince reluctantly agrees to marry but none of the eligible princesses strikes his fancy . . . and then he meets Prince Lee.
- *Mommy's Family* by Nancy Garden. 2004. Gr. K–3.
  When a classmate tells her, "no one has two mommies," Molly is upset and confused. But as her mommies and teacher help her understand that all families are different, she becomes proud of her own family.
- *Antonio's Card/La Tarjeta de Antonio* by Rigoberto Gonzalez. 2005. Gr. 2–5.
  With Mother's Day coming, Antonio has to decide what is important to him when his classmates make fun of the unusual appearance of his mother's partner, Leslie.
- *Daddy, Papa and Me* and *Mommy, Mama and Me* by Leslea Newman. 2009. Gr. Pre-K–1.
  This board book with rhyming text shows a toddler spending the day with his/her daddies or with her/his mommies.
- *In Our Mothers' House* by Patricia Polacco. 2009. Gr. 1–6.
  The oldest of three adopted children recalls their childhood with their mothers, Marmee and Meema.
- *A Tale of Two Daddies* by Vanita Oelschlager. 2010. Gr. 1–4.
  A young girl describes how her two daddies help her through her day.

REFERENCES

American Civil Liberties Union. (2017, March 6). *G.G. v. Gloucester County School Board*. Retrieved November 3, 2017. https://www.aclu.org/cases/gg-v-gloucester-county-school-board.

American Psychological Association. (2013). *Diagnostic and statistical manual of mental disorders (DSM-5)*, 5th ed. Arlington, VA: American Psychiatric Publishing.

American Psychological Association. (2017). *Resolution of gender and sexual orientation diversity in children and adolescents in schools*. Retrieved November 3, 2017. http://www.apa.org/about/policy/orientation-diversity.aspx.

Azzopardi-Lane, C., and Callus, A. (2015). Constructing sexual identities: People with intellectual disability talking about sexuality. *British Journal of Learning Disabilities*, 43(1): 32–37. DOI:10.1111/bld.12083.

Bedard, C., Hui, L. Z., and Zucker, K. J. (2010). Gender identity and sexual orientation in people with developmental disabilities. *Sexuality and Disability*, 28(3): 165–75. DOI:10.1007/s11195–010–9155-7.

Bryan, J. (2012). *From the dress-up corner to the senior prom: Navigating gender and sexuality diversity in pre-K-12 schools.* New York: Rowman & Littlefield Education.

Bryan, J. (2015). Beyond tomboys, sissies, and "that's so gay." Team Finch. Retrieved November 3, 2017. https://teamfinchconsultants.com/wp-content/uploads/2016/06/Beyond-Tomboys-Sissies-and-Thats-So-Gay-2-1-3.pdf.

Diamond, M. (2006). Biased-interaction theory of psychosexual development: "How does one know if one is male or female?" *Sex Roles*, 55: 589–600.

Dragowski, E. A., Scharrón-del Río, M. R., and Sandigorsky, A. L. (2011). Childhood gender identity . . . disorder? Developmental, cultural, and diagnostic concerns. *Journal of Counseling and Development*, 89(3): 360–66.

Drescher, J., and Pula, J. (2017). Expert Q and A: Gender Dysphoria. Retrieved November 3, 2017, from https://www.psychiatry.org/patients-families/gender-dysphoria/expert-qa on.

Freeman, J., and Knowles, K. (2012). Sex vs. gender: Cultural competence in health education research. *American Journal of Health Studies*, 27(2): 122–25.

Gender Spectrum. (2016). Retrieved November 3, 2017. https://www.genderspectrum.org/bathroomfaq/.

Jahoda, A., and Pownall, J. (2014). Sexual understanding, sources of information and social networks; the reports of young people with intellectual disabilities and their non-disabled peers. *Journal of Intellectual Disability Research*, 58(5): 430–41. DOI:10.1111/jir.12040.

Kothlow, K., and Chamberlain, K. (2012). *Disrupting heteronormativity in schools* (doctoral dissertation). Retrieved from ProQuest Dissertations and Theses. http://hdl.handle.net.libproxy. Lib.unc.edu/2429/42758.

Luyckx, K., Vansteenkiste, M., Goossens, L., and Duriez, B. (2009). Basic need satisfaction and identity formater: Bridging self-determination theory and process-oriented identity research. *Journal of Counseling Psychology*. DOI: 10.1037/a0015349.

Niles, G., and Harkins Monaco, E. A. (2017). Gender identity and sexual diversity: Supporting individuals with an intellectual or developmental disability. Manuscript submitted to *DADD Online Journal*.

Parekh, R. (2016). What Is Gender Dysphoria? Retrieved on November 3, 2017. https://www.psychiatry.org/patients-families/gender-dysphoria/what-is-gender-dysphoria.

Planned Parenthood (2017). Gender and gender identity. Retrieved November 3, 2017. https://www.plannedparenthood.org/learn/sexual-orientation-gender/gender-gender-identity#sthash.9xfuo4U7.dpuf.

Richards, C., and Barker, M. J. (2015). *The Palgrave handbook of the psychology of sexuality and gender*. New York: Palgrave MacMillan.

Sherer, I., Baum, J., Ehrensaft, D., and Rosenthal, S. M. (2015, January). Affirming gender: Caring for gender-atypical children and adolescents. *Contemporary Pediatrics*, 32(1): 16–19.

Vries, A., Steensma, T., Cohen-Kettenis, P., VanderLaan, D., and Zucker, K. (2016). Poor peer relations predict parent- and self-reported behavioral and emotional problems of adolescents with gender dysphoria: A cross-national, cross-clinic comparative analysis. *European Child and Adolescent Psychiatry*, 25(6): 579–88. DOI:10.1007/s00787-015-0764-7.

Chapter 8

Special Considerations: Group Homes and Residential Facilities

A young woman with an intellectual disability lives in a residential place-ment. Last week, the staff noticed she was scratching her vaginal area in public. Despite reminders that this is private behavior, the scratching contin-ued. The staff made an appointment with her primary care physician. Prior to engaging in the physical exam, the clinician asked questions to gather information on the patient's symptoms, sexual behaviors, and the patient's knowledge of safely engaging in sexual practices. The doctor learned that the patient has a boyfriend who also lives in the residential program, and once a week they watch movies in his room. They are sexually active during these weekly dates. The staff was unaware they were in a relationship, let alone the sexual activity.

The doctor expressed concern that this client may have contracted a sexu-ally transmitted infection (STI). She was also concerned that the patient was not aware of safe sexual practices, nor was the staff aware that two of their clients were sexually involved. The doctor asked the staff to put the following protocols in place:

- Discuss methods to sensitively approach sexual education and health and safety with their clients.
- Identify verbal or nonverbal strategies to identify safe sexual practices in the residential environment.
- Define risk factors for health conditions related to sexual activity.
- Outline techniques for tailoring health and wellness to the sexual needs of the clients in the residential placement.

SUMMARY

This chapter will cover the special considerations for those who work in group or residential homes. It will discuss training, differences between different providers, and the various institutional policies that may affect living conditions. The need for continued and continuous long-term sexual education is paramount, and for many of the individuals, no matter where they live, it is often neglected.

It is different from education in schools in that, as a part of group living arrangements and activities, there is often close proximity to others and frequent opportunities to spend unstructured (and sometimes unsupervised) time. There are many different types of residential living situations for individuals with intellectual disabilities and autism. This chapter will profile the most popular and provide suggested guidance for each; readers will be able to identify the following:

- Service providers for group homes and day programs for adults
  - who might be involved
  - educational background
  - training
  - in-services by experts
- Differences between different providers
- Living conditions and supervision
- Institutional policies
  - age-appropriate dating
  - legal Concerns
  - privacy
  - consent
  - relationships

TYPES OF RESIDENTIAL SETTINGS
AND SERVICES PROVIDED

Residential options for adults with intellectual disabilities and autism spectrum disorder typically address medical, behavioral, self-care, and/or daily living skill needs. Residential agencies offer graduated levels of assistance with options ranging from group homes to independent living with some supervision. Agencies provide services based on consumer needs and interests. Organizations that provide services vary widely in their staffing patterns, training, and ability to provide programming.

It is important to note that due to state wait-lists, group homes are now mostly populated by adults with the most severe cognitive, behavioral, physical, or medical needs. In addition, adults move to the top of the wait-list if there is a family crisis such as the death of parents or caregivers. Those with less severe impairments are more likely to remain at home with family or live in semi-independent settings.

A continuum of services was first conceptualized regarding the provision of special education services in the least restrictive environment (Deno 1970) and that has been the expectation and rule of law since then (Yell 2016). In 2001, Taylor similarly described a continuum of community integration describing residential settings:

Although there are exceptions, starting from the left of figure 8.1, the most restrictive residential settings are more medically oriented. The most restrictive settings include public and private institutions, nursing homes, and ICF/MR facilities (Taylor 2001). Institutions are typically defined as having sixteen or more residents. Included at this end of the continuum are also state hospital and correctional facilities that are designed to meet mental health and rehabilitation needs.

Residents of state institutions, residential schools, or treatment centers are clearly segregated from the mainstream community and have few opportunities for making independent decisions.

These settings often have strict rules of conduct regarding contact with others. Many of these settings are gender segregated with men's and women's units/wards. Some residents in correctional facilities have been perpetrators of sexual misconduct with charges ranging from public indecency to assault involving children or other adults with IDDs and ASDs.

Questions arise regarding whether the residents have been provided with education and support in learning acceptable social-sexual behaviors. For residents of these settings, basic sexuality education is needed. Education may include instruction and practice in topics like (1) public versus private settings, (2) understanding personal boundaries, (3) appropriate ways to express emotions, (4) who is and is not appropriate to engage in sexual behavior, (5) sexual abuse awareness, and (6) refusal skills. This type of instruction also needs to include helping the perpetrator to understand specifically why he or she has been incarcerated.

Although there are exceptions, at the most restrictive end of the continuum—nursing homes, ICF/MR facilities, private institutions and correctional facilities—services are often provided to those who have the most intense needs or those sometimes awaiting the transition to a less restrictive alternative.

The following is a description of the locations and the typical supports provided. We have also provided descriptive phrases for many of the locations regarding the specific issues related to sexual education for residents.

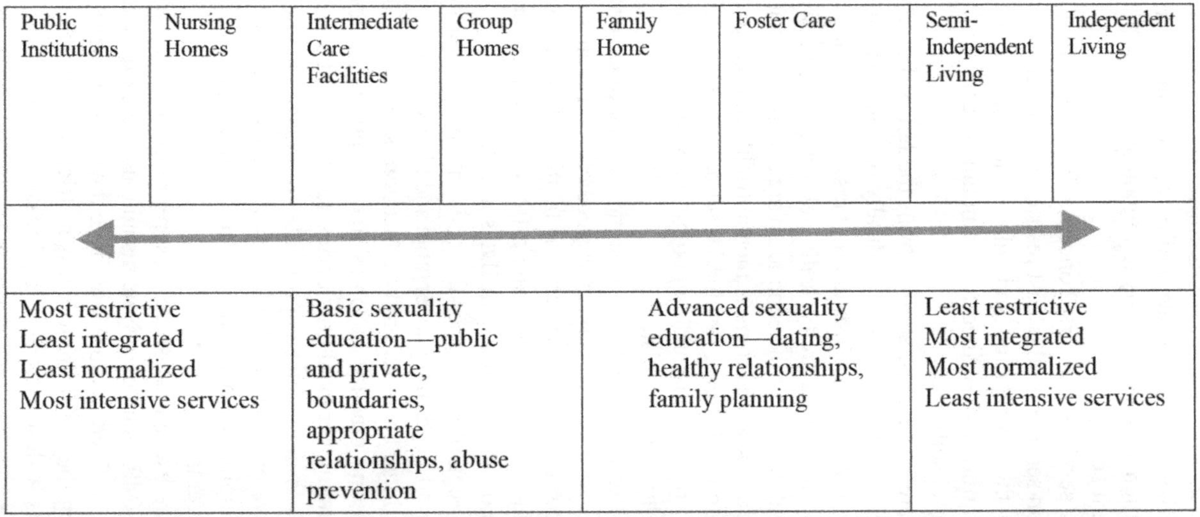

Public Institutions	Nursing Homes	Intermediate Care Facilities	Group Homes	Family Home	Foster Care	Semi-Independent Living	Independent Living
Most restrictive Least integrated Least normalized Most intensive services		Basic sexuality education—public and private, boundaries, appropriate relationships, abuse prevention		Advanced sexuality education—dating, healthy relationships, family planning		Least restrictive Most integrated Most normalized Least intensive services	

Figure 8.1   Continuum of residential options for adults with intellectual disabilities.
(Adapted from Taylor (2001), Figure 1, The Traditional Residential Continuum, 18.)

These are all generalizations, and the specific location where one works may be different (sometimes very different).

Most Restrictive: Gender Separate

Corrections institutions. There is often an issue of perpetrators. Individuals are there due to involvement with the legal system. The purpose of the correctional institutions is on incarceration and removing individuals who have problems with the law from society. The purpose of correctional institutions is not sexual education for individuals with IDDs and ASDs, so there is a distinct lack of knowledge about how to provide appropriate services for individuals.

Additionally, since the individuals involved in correctional institutions have typically been adjudicated as someone who violates the law and may be housed in close quarters with others, there are often issues related to socially accepted behaviors. This is not the ideal location for successful or intensive sexual education for individuals with IDDs or ASDs. Finally, correction institutions are infrequently used when a short-term emergency placement is warranted. An extensive search found no curriculum or materials related to sexuality education.

Hospitals. There is often very close control, often more for short term, as a means for addressing health or physical problems. The main purpose of a hospital is to address an individual's underlying concerns, be they physical or mental health. By nature they are intense and work to rule out other issues so as to address the health concern and to stabilize the individual.

This setting is also not conducive to providing appropriate instruction and supports to provide instruction related to sexual education for individuals with IDDs or ASDs. An extensive search found no curriculum or materials related to sexuality education.

Psychiatric treatment facilities. Like a hospital-based setting listed above, a psychiatric treatment facility often has a very specific purpose—that of helping an individual with very intensive psychiatric needs get and maintain control so as to function independently in the world. The problem is that psychiatric treatment facilities have been historically used to restrict individuals with IDDs and ASDs from society, further exacerbating stereotypes that they should be removed from the general population.

Individuals who become involved in psychiatric facilities may have maladaptive behaviors that may require intense supports and close control to assist in addressing the underlying mental health needs. An extensive search found no curriculum or materials related to sexuality education.

Halfway houses. All of the other living arrangements discussed in this section are very restrictive and have very specific focuses, be they correctional health or supports for psychiatric problems. This one is different as it is often viewed as a step between the intense needs of the above-listed locations and integration back into other living situations.

Depending on the halfway house and the needs demonstrated by the individuals, there may be partial community integration. Relationships can be tightly controlled. An extensive search found no curriculum or materials related to sexuality education.

These settings are usually seen as temporary placements for people with disabilities; however, in some cases, the period may be very much extended. For example, a person with a disability may be incarcerated for a serious crime or may have a chronic physical or mental illness. These cases may mean prolonged and/or sporadic placements in these restrictive environments. The availability of sexuality education in these settings depends upon the facility and on the administrators' perceptions of what is most important for the person with a disability at that particular time.

Homes

Parents or guardians homes. It is one of the most typical locations for individuals with IDD and ASD to live. It is very different from one location to another, so generalities are not applicable.

Foster homes. It is usually court appointed. Like parents or guardians homes, foster homes are very different from one location to another. They also can be very variable in terms of level of freedom in relationships. They may allow dating but are not usually going to have a private place to have sex while living in your parents' house.

Moderate Restrictions

Group homes and supervised apartments. These are gender segregated. Group homes may offer a little more independence and integration but vary in the amount of freedom residents are allowed to express in areas such as structuring and choosing activities, choosing friends outside the group home, and whether residents are allowed to date or have intimate relationships. They are often for individuals with good behavior, no trouble with authorities, and zero arrests.

Supervised apartments offer more freedom and choices than group homes or institutions. Support staff is available close by, but they only provide support, training in daily living skills, or recreational skills for a few hours a day. Residents typically live in a separate apartment with a roommate, as opposed to the group home model where all residents share common areas such as dining and leisure areas. Supervised apartments are typically gender mixed within the complex but not within the same apartment. An extensive search found little curriculum or materials related to sexuality education.

Fewer Restrictions

Supported living. It is like living in one's own apartment, could be mixed gender, and could have coupled relationship. Agencies may still impose some rules. It is variable. Living support training is a less restrictive option with the support worker visiting as needed to help with bill paying, shopping, and so on. This model provides a truly integrated residential situation, where the resident is living in the community independently but with a safety net.

Living support is very appealing for individuals with mild to moderate disabilities that desire independence but may need assistance. Many times, living support is made available after a resident has successfully proven competence in certain skill areas while living in a supervised apartment.

Least Restrictive

Independent living. It is living in one's own apartment with natural supports.

As you can see as we have profiled the various locations, we move from most restrictive to less restrictive and made generalities about each. However, what is evident is the lack of curriculums related to providing sexuality education for individuals with IDDs or ASDs. As was noted above, the need is clearly evident due to the long-term care needs along with the often close proximity of the living situations.

LIVING CONDITIONS AND SUPERVISION

As has been noted several times in other chapters, the biggest problem relates to perceptions of individuals with intellectual disabilities. It is important to understand the types of sexual offenses that are most common and why supervision is important. The most frequent sexual offenses reported in one study were indecent exposure, other minor offenses, and sexual assault of young girls (Day 1997).

Another nationwide study that surveyed 243 community agencies found that the most common sexual offenses were inappropriate sexual behavior in public (62.2 percent), sexual behaviors and stimulation that inappropriately involved others (42.6 percent), sexual activity involving minors (42.6 percent), and assaultive/nonconsensual sexual activity not involving minors (34.5 percent; Ward, Trigler, and Pfeiffer 2001). Another study found the most common sexual behaviors are those seen among people without intellectual disability—offenses against children, genital exposure, and rape (Murphy, Coleman, and Haynes 1983).

Safety and Regulations

It is very important to understand the institutional policies in place. Some prevent opportunities for expression, while others foster opportunities for individuals to receive education related to sexuality. There are often legal concerns—see the section on consent in chapter 10. One of the most important questions is whether the program participant/resident is their own legal guardian? Additionally, are there policies that prevent integration or prevent contact with others? Are there policies related to violation of rules? Can this lead to further segregation? Can it result in losing housing? Policies vary from location to location. It is imperative to understand the differences.

Supporting Relationships

It may be challenging for young adults in residential programs to start new friendships with like-minded people, as they may have difficulty finding peers who share interests and abilities. Individuals with IDDs and ASDs may be likely to look to the people around them within the programs as partners. It is essential then, for those living and working with people with IDDs and ASDs, to be educated in the importance of relationships and how to support their clients (Mirfin-Veitch 2003).

The residential staff assumes responsibility for residential policies, appropriate elements of development and safety, and typical privacy and decorum expectations that are considered the norm for adults without cognitive disabilities. Public, personal, and private behaviors are of primary importance, especially when considering residential policies. For example, if the staff is teaching that private acts must take place only in private places, staff must allow privacy for their clients for these acts as appropriate.

They must also address many other nuances of social relationships including but not limited to making and keeping friends, social compromise, perspective taking, asking for a date or a relationship, how to accept rejection, interpersonal communication skills, physical and social boundaries, and sexual health. Abuse prevention and focus on building healthy relationships are particularly critical, especially if the person with IDD or ASD does not have involvement with their family. Efforts to provide support and respect for a variety of relationships need to be created around the clients' senses of identity and their abilities to understand and communicate consent.

People with IDDs and ASDs experience challenges when navigating social norms, particularly when these social situations occur in their natural or home environments. That means they are working harder than most other people to organize and manage reciprocal relationships, let alone balancing romantic interests and social behaviors. It's important to remember this extra effort can increase stress or exacerbate behaviors for people with IDDs and ASDs, so helping clients take care of themselves is important. A number of different approaches can be applied, but the following guidelines in table 8.1 can help you get started:

Table 8.1 Recommendations to Help Clients Build Physical, Emotional, and Social Health

Help your clients . . .	*By supporting this . . .*
Take care of their physical health	• Getting proper sleep • Balancing a healthy diet • Teaching about nutrition • Exercise
Take care of their emotional health	• Provide ample therapeutic supports • Establish appropriate coping strategies • Encourage age-appropriate ways to address emotional well-being (individual or group counseling, role-plays, or watching TV shows/movies that depict social interactions and discussing them)
Take care of their social health	• Provide consistent support in navigating the social world (workplace, residential, community outings, etc.) • Facilitate access to and participation in activities in the community that are age-appropriate • Support and provide opportunities for varied social interaction

(LDA, n.d.)

Don't forget to honor the individual's individualism! This should especially include gender or sexual identity, personal preferences, and/or personal sexual or social needs.

CONCLUSION

It is with great disappointment that we report on the lack of curriculum related to sexuality education for one of the most important areas of the life of an individual with IDD or ASD. The variability and the other needs (physical or mental health) often prevent the focus on sexual expression. This may pose a long-term problem for individuals as they are seeking to not only be included but to participate in society as functioning adult.

RESOURCES

Chapter Books/Articles

Arlyn J. Roffman (2011). *Meeting the challenge of learning disabilities in adulthood.* Baltimore: Brookes Publishing Co.

National Center for Learning Disabilities, "Developing Social Skills and Relationships," http://www.ncld.org/parents-child-disabilities/social-emotional-skills/developing-social-skills-relationships.

National Center for Learning Disabilities, "Dr. Arlyn Roffman on Promoting Self-Awareness and Self-Acceptance in Teens," http://www.ncld.org/parents-child-disabilities/teens/dr-arlyn-roffman-promoting-self-awareness-self-acceptance-teens.

Reiff, H. (n.d). Social skills and adults with learning disabilities. Retrieved from http://www.ldonline.org/article/6010/.

Semrud-Clikeman, M., and Hynd, G. W. (1990). Right hemisphere dysfunction in nonverbal learning disabilities: Social, academic, and adaptive functioning in adults and children. *Psychological Bulletin*, 107(2): 196–209. http://dx.doi.org/10.1037/0033-2909.107.2.196.

Books

1. *Education for Life: Preparing Children to Meet Today's Challenges* by Donald Walters, published in 2004. This book does not have students with developmental disabilities as its focus and has a significant spiritual focus.
2. *Skills for Families, Skills for Life: How to Help Parents and Caregivers Meet the Challenges of Everyday Living*, by multiple authors, published in 2010. It has one chapter focusing on sexual education, but the main focus is independent living aspects. It does a good job of those components, though.
3. *The Everything Parent's Guide to Special Education: A Complete Step-by-Step Guide to Advocating for Your Child with Special Needs* by Amanda Morin, published in 2014. It covers the basics of special education and how to advocate for your child who has a disability.
4. *Sexuality and Relationship Education for Children and Adolescents with Autism Spectrum Disorders: A Professional's Guide to Understanding, Preventing . . . and Responding to Inappropriate Behaviours*, published in 2014, focuses solely on individuals with autism. It has good information and works to address the needs of individuals with developmental disabilities.
5. *Sexuality and Relationships in the Lives of People with Intellectual Disabilities*, by multiple authors, published in 2014. This book has a wealth of stories about individuals and by individuals with intellectual disabilities. It has great stories.
6. *Supporting Disabled People with Their Sexual Lives* by Tuppy Owens and Claire de Than, published in 2014. This book is more of a guide for people with disabilities than for others.
7. *When Young People with Intellectual Disabilities and Autism Hit Puberty: A Parents Q&A Guide to Health, Sexuality, and Relationships*, by Freddy Jackson Brown

and Sarah Brown, published in 2016. This book has a wealth of resources for parents in a question-and-answer format.

REFERENCES

Day, K. (1997). Clinical features and offense behavior of mentally retarded sex offenders: A review of research. *NADD Newsletter*, 14: 86–90.

Deno, E. (1970). Special education as developmental capital. *Exceptional Children,* 37: 229–37.

Mirfin-Veitch, Brigit (2003). *Relationships and adults with an intellectual disability: Review of the literature prepared for the National Advisory Committee on Health and Disability to inform its project on services for adults with an intellectual disability*. National Advisory Committee on Health and Disability.

Murphy, W., Coleman, E. and Haynes, M. (1983). Treatment and evaluation issues with the mentally retarded sex offender. In J. G. Greer and I. R. Stuart (Eds.), *The sexual aggressor: Current perspectives on treatment* (22–41). New York: Van Nostrand Reinhold.

Taylor, S. J. (2001). The continuum and current controversies in the USA. *Journal of Intellectual and Developmental Disability*, 26(1): 15–33.

Ward, K., Trigler, J., and Pfeiffer, K. (2001). Community services, issues, and service gaps for individuals with developmental disabilities who exhibit inappropriate sexual behaviors. *Mental Retardation*, 39(1): 11–19.

Yell, M. L. (2016). *The law and special education* (4th ed.). Upper Saddle River, NJ: Pearson.

Chapter 9

Similarities and Differences: ASD and IDD

SUMMARY

The characteristics of people with intellectual disabilities (IDDs) and autism spectrum disorders (ASDs) vary widely both within each category and between categories. Because of this variety, parents and educators know that an individual approach to transition to adulthood is preferred. Successful transition programs provide training and experience for students with disabilities (SWD) in the areas of work, postsecondary education, and community living. Though sexuality education falls in the category of successful transition to independent living in the community, many programs and school systems do not structurally address it as part of transition. Attaining successful intimate relationships with others is a goal that those without disabilities work toward. We should assume that those with IDDs and ASDs have the same interests in this general goal.

This chapter will highlight the following:

- general characteristics of those with IDD and ASD
- how these characteristics specifically affect sexuality and sexuality education for both groups
- the differences within each group based on functional levels
- the extra barriers faced by those with concurrent physical disabilities
- several scenarios for further writing and research

CHARACTERISTICS OF PEOPLE WITH ASDS

ASD is a neurodevelopmental disorder that impairs the child's ability to communicate and interact with others. It includes restricted and repetitive behaviors, interests, and activities (Mayo Clinic 2017). The term *spectrum* refers to the wide range of characteristics that may be present in any given individual that can affect social interaction, communication, behavior, and self-regulation. Severity is based on social communication impairments and the restrictive and repetitive nature of behaviors, as well as the ability to function independently.

Communication/social interaction: Appears not to hear; resists cuddling, prefers to play alone, retreats into own world; poor eye contact; delayed or no speech; social conversation deficits; conversation for requests or to "profess"; repetition without understanding the meaning; does not express emotions or feelings; appears unaware of others' feelings; reciprocal communication; and matching face to what is being communicated.

Patterns of behavior: Repetitive movements; routines or rituals, upset if unable to follow them; resistance to change; clumsiness; focuses on a specific part but may miss the whole when observing or listening; may have sensitivity to light or noise or touch; does not engage in imitative or make-believe play; overly focused interests; little or inconsistent eye contact; and struggles with daily living skills.

IQ can range from high to significantly below average. The CDC reports that 46 percent of children with ASDs have above-average IQ, but their ability to learn ranges widely. Children with ASDs tend to be strong visual learners. Age of diagnosis for high-functioning individuals may be a factor in ongoing success as adults. The characteristics of children with high-functioning ASDs may be missed or wrongly attributed by teachers and parents. This can cause delay in referral for diagnosis and special education support.

CHARACTERISTICS OF PEOPLE WITH IDDS

Those who fit the criteria for IDD display significant limitations both in intellectual functioning and in adaptive behavior (American Association on Intellectual or Developmental Disabilities 2017). A significant limitation in intellectual functioning translates to an IQ at or below 70 on a standardized intelligence scale; individual scores can range from not measurable to 70. Those with an IQ in this range have problems with memory, reading, writing, vocabulary, grammar, abstract thinking, generalization, logical problem solving, and social learning.

Adaptive behavior can be thought of as practical intelligence or the ability to solve every day problems (Hallahan, Kauffman, and Pullen 2015). These problems can include selecting appropriate clothes, accessing transportation, soft job skills, interacting with authority, making friends, communication, bathing, dressing, preparing food, safety concerns, living independently, maintaining employment, and others.

Those with IDDs generally do not meet developmental milestones for children, such as babbling, speaking, crawling, walking, at the same time period as typically developing children. They may have a limited understanding right from wrong and trouble managing frustration or self-regulation. People with IDDs can have deficits in metacognition and the ability to select strategies to solve a problem, try a strategy, and evaluate its effectiveness. Those with IDDs tend to be more gullible than typically developing children and adults.

SIMILARITIES BETWEEN GROUPS AND SEXUALITY IMPLICATIONS

The similarities between IDD and ASD characteristics match up for different subgroups within the two populations. The IQ and functional range within ASD overlaps and can greatly exceed that of those with IDD; however, there is overlap between those with moderate and mild IDD and some of those with ASD. For example, higher-functioning people with IDDs can live independently, some with and some without supervision; there are many people with ASDs who live independently.

Table 9.1 shows shared characteristics of the two groups that affect healthy sexual development:

Table 9.1   Healthy Sexual Development

Individual's need to understand . . .	By developing the following . . .
• Positive communication about sexual encounters • Reciprocity in intimate relationships both emotionally and sexually • Application of sexual education ideas after they have been learned • Concern that the partner has really consented • When to talk about sex and with whom • Birth control • Negative perceptions about sex • Misinformation learned from uninformed others • Personal incomplete learning about sexuality • Behavior that leads to social isolation	• Appropriate public and private interactions with partners • Ability to navigate mass media portrayals of sex and/or access to pornography and the related unrealistic ideal of sexual encounters. • Self-advocacy and self-awareness • Ability to tolerate frustration • Ability to navigate others' ideas and comfort level with sexuality and sexuality education • Seek out health and safety protocols • Seek out opportunities to reinforce learning • Behavior that negates social isolation (social pragmatics, self-determination, and emotional management)

An important consideration for those with either IDDs or ASDs is the amount and quality of social interactions they have over their childhood and adolescence. Socializing with potential partners is a step that can lead to healthy sexual relationships. Both groups can be socially isolated from others with a similar disorder and those with no disabilities. The isolation can be a result of the characteristics of the disabilities.

For individuals with ASD specifically, the reciprocal nature of social interaction is not always fully developed. This can be as simple as misunderstanding the conventions of communication: one-person talks, the other listens, reverse and repeat. Individuals with IDDs may have a misconception about the nature or depth of a relationship; they may mistake casual social interactions as close friendship that can lead to more intimate relationships.

Regardless of the cause, individuals with either IDDs or ASDs need to be helped to have positive social interactions with others with and without disabilities throughout their childhood and adolescence and into adulthood in order to develop healthy future sexual relationships.

Another shared set of characteristics between the two groups is their ability to learn and benefit from learning. For people with IDD, a deficit in learning is part of the definition of the disorder; they do not learn as efficiently as typically developing students; they are likely to understand concrete concepts but struggle with abstraction and have difficulty generalizing learned information to other contexts.

Those with ASDs too have been found to have rigid or stereotyped thinking where new information is less likely to be assimilated if it does not fit with an existing idea. People with ASDs also have trouble generalizing something learned in one context to another, particularly less structured, context. Both groups have trouble with social or casual learning within the social context—arguably, the primary means for typically developing peers to gather information about sexuality. For these reasons, sexuality education instruction needs to be geared directly to the learning strengths of these groups. This will require different approaches for different individuals but in general visual instruction that includes role-play with reinforcement is indicated.

Both groups will benefit from instruction in self-regulation to manage sexual development. They need help with the metacognitive process of problem solving related to sexual development. Typically, self-regulation is thought of as a system in which a learner attempts to solve a problem by selecting a strategy, implementing the strategy, receiving feedback about the strategy, and then adapting and attempting a new strategy.

Teachers and parents can intervene in self-regulation by providing co-regulation, in particular, helping with feedback about how effective a particular strategy was in reaching the intended goal. For example, teachers can ask a boy with ASD if hanging out watching field hockey practice was an effective means to talking with a girl on the field hockey squad and how this might be perceived by others. This conversation could be further extended to help the student with generalization and opportunities to practice a new idea.

DIFFERENCES BETWEEN GROUPS
AND SEXUALITY IMPLICATIONS

There are several specific differences between the characteristics of those with IDDs and ASDs. An important one for some people with ASD is the difference in perceptions of sensory input; they may be overly sensitive to touch. Those with hypersensitivity to touch are less likely to want to be touched in presexual ways as a child, for example, a massage or hug from a parent. These early types of touch can later be part of how sexual partners communicate; those with this specific characteristic miss out on learning these early stages.

Some communication deficits are specific to those with ASDs. Many children with ASDs lack communicative intent, the desire to communicate for social purposes, and with joint attention, the process where one individual communicates about a stimulus through nonverbal means (Hallahan et al. 2015). Some people with ASDs fail to understand how others feel in general and how others feel about things that they do.

As described elsewhere in this text, communication is particularly important for healthy intimate and sexual relationships. Those with ASDs who have severe communication deficits can become more isolated from others, and this isolation contributes to delayed socialization. Since socialization is part of healthy sexual development, communication deficits negatively affect sexual development.

A subset of those with ASDs also has anxiety and other mental health concerns. As described above, communication deficits can lead to social isolation. People with ASDs also often have repetitive behavior and catastrophic reactions to seemingly small events or change. These behaviors too can lead to social isolation and a misperception by others that people with ASDs prefer to be alone.

People with IDDs have other characteristics that are specific to them that affect their ability to learn about and participate in healthy sexuality. People with IDDs are more likely to be gullible than their typically developing peers. Gullibility is the tendency to believe in something that is likely false (Hallahan et al. 2015). This characteristic opens people with IDDs up for potential problems from simple teasing to participating in criminal activity to victimization. They are less likely to be able to spot others who intend to do them harm; for this reason, the rates of sexual abuse for people with IDDs are higher than those of the average population.

Some people with IDDs tend to act more childlike or to behave in the way a child does even when they are no longer children. For example, some people with IDDs may be overly affectionate to hug new acquaintances or strangers. This obviously sends a mixed signal to others. Alternatively, people with IDDs are likely to develop physically before their cognitive ability can fully develop; related to sexuality, they may appear to be physically ready for an intimate or sexual relationship; however, their cognitive and social ability to negotiate the relationship is delayed.

SPECIAL CONSIDERATIONS FOR THOSE WITH LOW IQ AND/OR FUNCTIONING LEVELS

The following characteristics are shared by those with IDDs and ASDs who have low IQ or functioning levels:

- ability to understand sexual education concepts beyond the concrete
- access to consenting partners if they live at home or in a facility
- others' perceptions of their rights to have sexual relationships
- increased victimization due to not understanding who is a friend and who is not
- inappropriate touching of others and self in public
- more likely to live in an institution
- may have trouble with cause and effect—their actions may actually push away a potential partner

One strong suggestion that we have made elsewhere in this text is for people with IDDs and ASDs to have ongoing and consistent instruction in sexuality education that includes constructive feedback from a trusted person. This may be particularly problematic for those with more severe characteristics of both disorders due to staff turnover and poor training. This can lead to partial instruction or no instruction at all in some areas of the curriculum. The other consideration for these students is that they may live with a parent or guardian who is their primary interpreter of the world at large. If that individual is not trained or interested in teaching sexuality education, the adolescent or young adult will not have access to it.

SPECIAL CONSIDERATIONS FOR THOSE WITH ASD OR IDD AND PHYSICAL DISABILITIES

For individuals with either ASDs or IDDs and physical disabilities, there are other barriers to intimate relations. Some physical disabilities directly affect sexual functioning and may preclude traditional sexual relationships. Others with physical disabilities require assistance in moving and transferring. These types of physical disabilities may limit potential partners to those who can help with transfers. As with others with ASDs or IDDs, limited social interactions and early presexual relationships will affect mature sexual relationships. Individuals with physical disabilities are particularly vulnerable to abuse by others.

SCENARIOS

1. Bob is a fifty-five-year-old man with IDD who lives in a residential facility with two other consumers and a rotating staff of live-in house parents. Since Bob uses a wheelchair and falls frequently, his service plan calls for the staff to keep him in visual proximity when he is awake. The staff has complained to their supervisor that Bob regularly masturbates in his bedroom with the door open.

   a. Name several solutions that take into consideration both Bob and the staff's concerns.
   b. Would you have different concerns if Bob was twenty-one instead of fifty-five?

2. Mary is an eighteen-year-old girl with Down syndrome. She is attracted to her twenty-two-year-old day program manager. She has shared with other staff that she finds him attractive, calls out his name loudly from across the day program work room when he arrives, comments about the clothes he wears, and asks him what he is doing on the weekend.

   a. What concerns do you have for Mary and the program manager?
   b. What, if anything, should the program manager say to Mary? Should this type of interaction be documented?

3. Bill is a nineteen-year-old student with ASD who has been dating Sue, a seventeen-year-old girl with ASD who is in his class. The two exchanged sexually explicit photos through their iPhones. Sue's mother monitors her phone usage and discovered the pictures.

   a. Examine your local school district policy about this type of interaction. How does it apply in this situation?
   b. In what ways do the students' disabilities interact with the policy? Should their disability characteristics be considered?

4. Doug is a sixteen-year-old boy with IDD and cerebral palsy. He uses a wheelchair to get around and needs to be driven when he leaves the home.

His mother buys his clothes and anything else he needs. Recently, Doug asked a male case manager to buy him some Vaseline in order to masturbate.

    a. Should the case manager honor Doug's request? If he does so, should he ask or inform Doug's mother?

    b. If you were the case manager, would you consider any other steps now that Doug has broached the topic?

5. Sue is a twenty-three-year-old woman with ASD who has recently moved into a supervised apartment with a roommate that is managed by a local agency. The agency does not provide 24/7 supervision of this apartment complex; in fact this apartment is one of two within the building that is managed for young adults with disabilities, the rest are rented out to the public in general. Sue's roommate reported to the case manager that Sue has been sleeping with one of the nondisabled residents of the building.

    a. How does this situation compare to that of any typically developing roommates with a boyfriend sleeping over?

    b. If you were the parent or guardian of Sue or her roommate, what concerns or actions might you consider?

CONCLUSION

Characterizing any group or subgroup is a difficult task. Within a given group there is wide variation. This is clearly the case for those with IDDs and ASDs. This chapter offered a general characterization based on the groups as a whole; anyone who knows individuals with either disability can identify individuals who do not exactly fit with these general descriptions.

Both groups vary by intellectual capacity, functional skills, and interest in socialization, independence, and more. In addition, this chapter highlighted deficits inherent in individuals who meet the diagnostic criteria for each disability; however, individuals with either diagnosis have many other characteristics and abilities that are not included here.

REFERENCES

American Association on Intellectual and Developmental Disabilities. (2017). Retrieved November 3, 2017. http://aaidd.org/intellectual-disability/definition#. WWuZxIqQyb8.

Autism Spectrum Disorder. National Institute of Mental Health. Retrieved, June 6, 2017. https://www.nimh.nih.gov/health/topics/autism-spectrum-disorders-asd/ index.shtml.

Hallahan, D., Kauffman, J. M., and Pullen, P. C. (2015). *Exceptional learners: An introduction to special education*, 13th ed. Boston, MA: Pearson.

Mayo Clinic (2017). Diseases and conditions: Autism spectrum disorder. Retrieved November 3, 2017, from http://www.mayoclinic.org/diseases-conditions/autism-spectrum-disorder/basics/definition/con-20021148.

Chapter 10

Just Say No (or Yes): Ethics

"Who gets to say whether I can learn about or have sex?"

Mary is twenty-one years old with an IQ of 65 who has intellectual disabilities. She has stated that she wants a boyfriend. Mary's family does what they can to prevent her from engaging with men because they fear Mary will be exploited or coerced into having sex. Recently, Mary has become interested in dating a young man from a college access program she attends at the local community college. He has a diagnosis of autism. Are there ethical issues regarding Mary developing an intimate relationship with this young man?

Mary also sees many attractive men on campus who are not in her program. She would like to flirt with them and get to know them better, but wonders whether they would be interested in her because of her disability. Are there ethical issues regarding Mary developing an intimate relationship with any of these men? Mary's family is against her developing any kind of intimate relationship. Are there ethical issues regarding what professionals in her program need to consider? Would the ethical issues be different if Mary was seventeen years old? What about if she was fifteen years old?

SUMMARY

For decades, people with intellectual disabilities and/or developmental disabilities have been thought to be asexual, having no need for loving and fulfilling relationships with others. Individual rights to sexuality, which is essential to human health and well-being, have been denied. This loss has negatively affected people with intellectual disabilities in gender identity, friendships, self-esteem, body image and awareness, emotional growth, and social behavior.

People with intellectual or developmental disabilities frequently lack access to appropriate sex education in schools and other settings. At the same time, some individuals may engage in sexual activity as a result of poor options, manipulation, loneliness, or physical force rather than as an expression of their sexuality (AAIDD 2013, 1).

After reading this chapter, readers will be able to define:

- protection
- capacity—consent to sex education, ethical duty to provide sex education
- capacity—consent to sexual relationships
- supported or substituted consent
- ethical issues involving protectionism
- legal guardianship
- consent and who can consent
- the elements of informed consent

ETHICAL ISSUES IN SEXUALITY EDUCATION

Historically, the stereotypes have been that individuals with IDDs and ASDs are eternal children with no sexual feelings, or they are sexual time bombs driven by animal instincts that pose a danger to others. These thoughts about individuals with IDDs and ASDs have influenced policies and practices regarding sexuality education for the past century (and maybe longer) (Doyle 2010; Herring 2012). Relationships have been inhibited or prevented under the assumption that people with IDDs would "not want to engage in sexual relationships, or could not do so in a meaningful way" (Herring 2012).

The concept of mental age can be misleading for parents and professionals leading them to believe that a young person with IDD or ASD is a five-year-old trapped in an adult body, living in a state of perpetual childhood never fully to enter adult status. However, adolescents and adults with IDDs and ASDs are not children; they do not have the same thoughts, feelings, and desires of children, and they do not live in a vacuum where images of sexuality and relationships have been filtered out. Nevertheless, attempts to control the sexual aspects of their lives have been made in the name of protectionism (Rojas 2014). For people with IDD, this has meant that a "fundamental part of their lives has been condemned to oblivion" (56).

Another assumption is that if young people with IDDs and ASDs are not protected *from* sexuality education, the mere talk about sex will awaken the dormant flames of desire and unleash a powerful destructive force that must be controlled. Although this may sound dramatic, control over sexual content and contact is merely one more step in a series of events controlled by others throughout the lives of people with IDDs and ASDs. The issue then becomes, if others have controlled so many aspects of one's life, how does one develop the ability to make decisions, especially decisions about one's own body and relationships with others?

We cannot discount the fact that many individuals with IDDs have been exploited and coerced into sexual relationships making protection from sexual predators morally, ethically, and legally of utmost importance (refer to chapter 1 and elsewhere in the book where there is a discussion of abuse). But, problems exist within a paternalistic protection/control point of view.

First, sexuality is more than sexual acts. Sexuality includes one's identity and thus how we see the world. Second, if we view people with IDDs as capable of learning and growing, adopting an overly restrictive approach preventing education about relationships that can enhance quality of life would be unethical. Third, a protection point of view goes against efforts to include more people with IDDs and ASDs in more inclusive school and community environments. Therefore, we need to view skills needed *in* these environments rather than protection *from* inclusive environments. According to Leicester and Cooke (2001), there may be a fine line between freedom and the need for protecting the most vulnerable adults in our society, but "their adult status surely permits them the dignity of an assumption of freedom within a framework of protection" (185).

Position Statement

According to a joint position statement of AAIDD and the Arc (AAIDD 2013), individuals with IDDs have a right to:

- sexual expression and education, reflective of their own cultural, religious and moral values and of social responsibility;
- individualized education and information to encourage informed decision-making, including education about such issues as reproduction, marriage and family life, abstinence, safe sexual practices, sexual orientation, sexual abuse, and sexually transmitted diseases; and
- protection from sexual harassment and from physical, sexual, and emotional abuse. (1)

Perhaps the first and foremost issue in sexuality education for students with IDDs and ASDs is consent. Who gets to consent to sexuality education? Who gets to consent to sexual relations?

ETHICS OF CONSENT AND SUPPORT

There is no internationally accepted definition of legal capacity. The need for understanding capacity reflects an individual's ability to make decisions that are binding.

Legal capacity is a particularly challenging and complex issue because it affects all areas of life, including where to live, whether and whom to marry, signing an employment contracts, having property, or casting a vote. The right to legal capacity is, therefore, closely entwined with equality and non-discrimination. At the center of this discussion is a person, and there needs to be discussions related to the implications for legal capacity legislation and its implementation for each individual.

There are two main types of considerations relating to capacity:

1. *Supported decision making*: This is where a support person enables a person with a disability to take and communicate decisions with respect to personal or legal matters. With supported decision making, the presumption is always in favor of the person with a disability who will be affected by the decision. The individual is the decision maker; the support person explains the issues, when necessary, and interprets the signs and preferences of the individual. Even when an individual with a disability requires total support, the support person should enable that person to exercise their legal capacity to the greatest extent possible, according to the latter's wishes and/or best interests.
2. *Substituted decision making*: This is where the legal representative, guardian, or tutor has court-authorized power to make decisions on behalf of the individual without necessarily having to demonstrate those decisions are in the individual's best interest or according to his or her wishes.

Additionally, there is a wide range of different terms used to discuss the issues surrounding legal capacity, in particular issues involving who is legally empowered to make decisions on another's behalf. The loss of legal capacity is, for example, distinct from the introduction of a protective measure that refers to the placement of an individual under guardianship and not to the loss of the person's legal capacity. Under guardianship, a legal representative makes binding decisions for the person placed under a protective measure. This is known as substituted decision making.

There is a difference between formal and informal restrictions on decision making. Formal restrictions of legal capacity are those in which an individual loses his or her power to make decisions recognized by law, wholly or in part, because of legal measures. This usually involves a court decision to deprive someone of his or her legal capacity, followed by the appointment of a guardian who makes legally binding decisions on his or her behalf.

Informal restrictions of legal capacity are often independent of any formal legal measure. They include factors and practices restricting the ability of a person to make decisions about his or her life. They are based on the assumption that persons with disabilities cannot make decisions for themselves because they do not understand the likely consequences of their actions, and it is therefore in their best interest if decisions are made on their behalf.

Guardianship

During the past forty years, society has become more aware of the capabilities of people with intellectual disabilities and their entitlement to basic human and legal rights (AAIDD 2013). With the growth of knowledge in the field of IDD and ASD and the development of advocacy groups, the public awakened to the fact that people with IDDs have long been denied full citizenship status guaranteed them by the Constitution (Shogren and Wehmeyer 2017).

This awareness has resulted in judicial decisions and legislative mandates, which seek to correct past deficiencies. There are still, however, areas of the law-requiring revision to reflect the change in attitudes and to ensure that theoretical legal victories are established in practice.

To do this, statutes should be revised, so people with varying levels of IDDs and ASDs are allowed to live as independently as they are able. To achieve this goal, legislators and members of the legal community must become aware of the nature of IDD and ASD, consider the personhood of each individual, and devise a legal framework with flexibility enough to accommodate the individual.

People with IDDs and ASDs have historically lost their individual identity to the generalizations of the condition. Once a person is known to have IDD or ASD, general incompetency has been assumed with little or no investigation of his or her actual capabilities.

A change in thinking has evolved among professionals in the field of IDD and ASD based on an increase in knowledge and the development of advocacy groups. It is now believed that assessment should begin with actual capabilities of the person with IDD and ASD before consideration of any of the general manifestations of the disability. This is required because there is a wide range of abilities, which will be affected by individual personality traits. Greater awareness of the range and nature of IDD and ASD is required by all professions to ensure the treatment or services provided are based on the needs of the individual and are not diluted by generalities of the condition.

Guardianship may be viewed as a mechanism of control or as a device to support the individual. The way it is viewed is significant when the adult with IDD or ASD is given more opportunity to make choices. If society deals with IDD and ASD by broad strokes and lacking individualization, it exercises maximum control in that form. Guardianship, if used at all, is often invoked only when there are considerable assets to manage.

In contrast, integration of citizens with IDDs and ASDs into society is characterized by choices and opportunities for all citizens and presents more significant and difficult questions concerning the proper use of guardianship. If community-based services are available to assist, guardianship should be viewed as a mechanism of support for the individual in making his or her own choices. A totally supportive structure of community-based services would drastically reduce the need to use guardianship at all.

In our society, however, guardianship is indispensable in the process of allowing an individual's access to society. It enables the person with IDD to be guided in areas where assistance is needed and would otherwise be unable to participate due to his inability to contact and evaluate existing community services.

Consent

Young people with IDDs need comprehensive sexuality education before they can provide informed consent. Sexuality education must provide information about building healthy relationships in addition to biological factors of maturation and physical sexual actions. According to Carmody and Ovenden (2013), young people need comprehensive education that covers sex, gender, and sexuality, as well as encouraging "verbal negotiation in everyday sexual encounters, to ensure consensual sexual experiences" (795).

Current best practice in sexuality education has shifted away from "moral-panic" approaches to approaches that recognize the agency of young people and enable them to negotiate ethical sexual lives (Carmody and Ovenden 2013).

The following are factors influencing changing views from protection/prevention to consent and support:

- Increased acknowledgment that many people with IDs can give consent to sexual relations (Leicester and Cooke 2002).
- With more community integration, there is less professional control, thus focus is to prevent abuse and unhealthy relationships rather than preventing relationships per se.
- Increased acknowledgment of the importance of human rights (Evans and Rodgers 2000).

Consent to Sexual Relations

Individuals may lack capacity to make some decisions but not to make others (Herring 2012). So does the individual have the capacity to give consent to sexual relations? The capacity to consent is situation- and person-specific. The individual needs to (a) understand the information relevant to the decision, (b) retain that information, (c) use or weigh that information in the process of making the decision, or (d) communicate his decision (Herring 2012).

What do we ask to determine capacity? Most court cases have used a medical model focusing on capacity to understanding the physical act, health risks, and consequences such as pregnancy or contracting an STI (Herring 2012).

What about the capacity to understand the emotional risks? The circumstances surrounding the sexual act must be considered. How was the encounter negotiated? Are there steps taken to ensure it was an act respecting their mutual interests (Herring 2012)? Does Mary in the above case understand something as subtle as level of commitment to the relationship? Understand whether she is being lied to? Understanding the difference between someone being tender and someone being exploitative? Is she consenting to a sexual act or a wider relational and social meaning (Herring 2012)?

With whom? There are some special circumstances of consent; for example, sex with one in position of power is determined exploitative. It is clear that sexual relations with a boss/supervisor, a caregiver, doctor/psychologist are not acceptable. But what about sexual activity between two people with IDDs?

In 2002, Spiecker and Steutel asked the question: is sex between adults with mildly or moderate ID morally permissible and, if at all, under what conditions? They noted that a distinctive characteristic of ID is practical rationality, which is the "capacity of determining and weighing the pros and cons of different actions one might perform under the circumstances, with the intention of determining which alternative is the right, most desirable or virtuous one" (160).

Individuals with IDs lack the deliberative capacity to think of long-term welfare of self or others, and they lack the practical rationality implied in adult status. This is why they are "permanently dependent on the paternalistic guidance and moral supervision of adult caregivers" (162).

> If valid consent is taken as a necessary condition of moral permissibility, many cases of sexual interaction between people with mental retardation should be deemed morally wrong, not because they are coerced or deceived, but because their capacities of judgement are deficient. (164)

Spiecker and Steutel's (2002) conclusion was that sexual interaction between people with IDDs is only morally permissible under adult supervision with the permission of caregivers.

Stephen Greenspan (2002) countered Spieker and Steutel's argument by stating that giving caregiver's substitutive consent and control over the *presumed incompetents* based on their best interest perpetuates the eternal child stereotype. This approach denies people with IDs the opportunity to make and learn from their mistakes. Another problem may involve which caregiver was in charge. One caregiver may allow sex and another may not.

The following is a discussion about the age of consent and issues related to mandated reporting:

1. State Laws—Age of Consent

a. Legal guardianship
   nj.gov/humanservices/ddd/services/guardianship

In a study conducted by O'Callaghan and Murphy (2007), about one-quarter of the participants with IDs were aware of the legal age of consent. Half either did not know whether they were allowed to have sex by law or thought that they were not allowed. One-third thought they were not allowed to get married by law, and 40 percent thought they were not allowed by law to decide about getting an abortion. When asked if there were special laws protecting people with IDs from abuse, most knew there were laws but did not know what they were. Half said that people with IDDs could not make proper decisions about having sexual relationships.

2. Responsibilities of Caregivers

a. Mandated reporting

A criticism of mandated reporting is that it produces numerous unsubstantiated reports and, therefore, increases workload for child protective services, wasting resources, and reducing the quality of service given to known deserving individuals with disabilities and their families (Schormans and Sobsey 2017). Without a system of mandated reporting, however, a society will be less able to protect vulnerable populations, because many cases of abuse and neglect will not come to the attention of the appropriate agencies. The most serious problem in mandated reporting appears to not be with reporting but with the responses.

If there was not a system where those who have disabilities may be abused, many and perhaps most cases will remain hidden. A society with mandated reporting will have more cases of abuse and neglect brought to the attention of authorities than will a society with no such system. Even so, many agree that legislation, reporter training, and public education should more clearly define what should and should not be reported.

Mandated reporters should receive thorough training (Crawford 2014), especially as it relates to individuals with disabilities. Methods of intake, screening, and assessment may be refined, and personnel can become more skilled (Schormans and Sobsey 2017).

The most significant problems are not with mandated reporting but with responses.

Mandated reporting produces more referrals, a proportion of which are not substantiated, which requires resources to screen, assess, and investigate, and this may distract overburdened personnel from known cases. However, this is not an argument against mandated reporting but against insufficient resourcing, perhaps ineffective reporter training and practice, less than optimum screening, and vague reporting laws.

There are problems of inadequate resources (Finkelhor 2005) and still developing methods of screening (Besharov 2005) and assessment. Mandated reporting is separate from the responses of child protective agencies. The task of these agencies is to develop sound policy and culture and to respond appropriately after referral.

Mandated reporting enables economic and social benefits far outweighing disadvantages.

Abuse and neglect cause sufficient economic and social cost to justify, if not demand, government responses. Calculating precise economic costs is not possible, and there is not yet a reliable body of evidence about the costs or the cost-effectiveness of prevention and intervention programs. Yet studies do indicate substantial economic costs (Crawford 2014) and suggest ongoing efforts to improve prevention, case finding, and intervention are fiscally imperative.

Society must not ignore wrongs committed by adults against individuals with disabilities. Law must treat people with respect and dignity, listen to their lived experience, and protect aspects of personal, family, and community life that maintain dignity (Brown, Radford, and Wehmeyer 2017). Philosopher John Stuart Mill identified the family sphere as the most important domain requiring the state control to prevent abuse of power (1998, 116).

Notions of parental liberty should not be unduly privileged over children's rights to personal security. That history and custom has left adults' treatment of children untended is no reason to still devalue children's liberty.

The principles that motivated mandated reporting originally are even more important today. True, the first laws were intended for an imagined several hundred cases of physical abuse. Yet, the purpose of those laws, then as now, was to bring cases of severe abuse to the attention of authorities because otherwise they would have remained hidden. We now know the number of cases is greater, the costs are extensive, and actions taken early in life can be highly beneficial.

The nature and efficacy of the system responding to reports are critical but separate challenges. Even with a good system of mandated reporting, many children's experience will go undetected. Without it, and without a proven alternative, many thousands more children will be left to suffer, incurring even more health and economic costs.

CONCLUSION

Teachers and service providers for people with IDDs and ASDs face ethical questions on a daily basis around the ideas of sexuality education and sexual relations. For example, special education teachers are mandated to prepare SWD to transition to adulthood. Many teachers and service providers believe that sexuality education should be part of that transition and that students and adults with IDDs and ASDs will engage in sexual relations.

However, families and some school districts hold different beliefs about these same students; that is, SWD should not have sexual education or any sexual relations. Some of this perspective stems from families' cultural or religious beliefs about sexuality education or from school board policy for all students in a district. Some of this perspective, as has been discussed above, comes from the natural impulse to protect students with IDDs and ASDs.

In the classroom or during down time at school, students with IDDs and ASDs have access to potential sexual partners and make attempts to flirt, develop relationships, or touch. Teachers in this situation, and service providers in the community, have a teaching opportunity when they witness these natural stages of sexual development. Teachers and service providers need to first ensure the safety of all students in their care. Their next steps can either be perceived as subversive or developmentally supportive by reacting with a mini sexual-education lesson or by simply separating students.

As with other ethical dilemmas, there is no hard correct answer to this one. Teachers and service providers not only need to honor the wishes of the families, but they also need to value the individual's sexual development. As mentioned elsewhere in this text, frank and frequent communication between all parties is strongly recommended.

Internet Resources

State policies on sex education:

- ncsl.org/research/health/state-policies-on-sex-education-in-schools.aspx
- ecs.org/clearinghouse/73/09/7309.pdf

Age of consent by state:

- legalmatch.com/law-library/article/age-of-consent-by-state

Consent regarding educational program:

- SPIN parent guide:
  spinhawaii.org/education-parent-guide/planning-for-transitions

Decisional capacity

Decisional capacity refers to an adult student being able to understand, reason, and act on his or her own behalf. If the student lacks decisional capacity, it means they are unable to provide informed *consent* for their educational program. Some parents will opt to become their child's legal guardian. This requires going to court and having a judge declare your child legally incompetent to make certain decisions for him- or herself. Another option that doesn't require legal action is to become your child's educational representative for special education purposes. All that is required is a written statement by a qualified professional (e.g., a physician, psychologist, psychiatrist, a representative from the Developmental Disabilities Division) that your child lacks decisional capacity due to his or her disability.

REFERENCES

American Association of Intellectual and Developmental Disabilities (AAIDD). (2013). Sexuality: Joint Position Statement of AAIDD and the Arc. https://aaidd. org/news-policy/policy/position-statements/sexuality.

Besharov, D. (2005). Overreporting and underreporting of child abuse and neglect are twin problems. In D. Loseke, R. Gelles, and M. Cavanaugh (Eds.), *Current controversies on family violence* (2nd ed., 285–98). Thousand Oaks, CA: Sage.

Brown, I., Radford, J. P., and Wehmeyer, M. L. (2017). Historical overview of intellectual and developmental disabilities. In M. L. Wehmeyer, I. Brown, M. Percey, K. A. Shogren, and W. L. A. Fung (Eds.), *A comprehensive guide to intellectual and developmental disabilities* (2nd ed., 19–34). Baltimore, MD: Paul H. Brookes Publishing Co.

Carmody, M., and Ovenden, G. (2013). Putting ethical sex into practice: Sexual negotiation, gender and citizenship in the lives of young women and men. *Journal of Youth Studies*, 16(6): 792–807.

Crawford, D. (2014). *Assessment of staff perception of sexual behavior among persons with intellectual and developmental disabilities* (Dissertation at the Massachusetts School of Professional Psychology).

Doyle, S. (2010). The notion of consent to sexual activity for persons with mental disabilities. *Liverpool Law Review*, 31(2): 111–35. DOI: 10.1007/s10991-010-9076-7.

Evans, A., and Rodgers, M.E. (2000). Protection for whom?: The right to a sexual or intimate relationship. *Journal of Intellectual Disabilities*, 4(3): 237–45.

Finkelhor, D. (2005). The main problem is underreporting child abuse and neglect. In D. Loseke, R. Gelles, and M. Cavanaugh (Eds.), *Current controversies on family violence* (2nd ed., 299–310). Thousand Oaks, CA: Sage.

Greenspan, S. (2002). A sex police for adults with "mental retardation"? Comment on Spiecker and Steutel. *Journal of Moral Education*, 31(2): 171–79. DOI: 10.1080/03057240220143278.

Herring, J. (2012). Mental disability and capacity to consent to sex: A local authority v H[2012] EWHC 49 (COP). *Journal of Social Welfare and Family Law*, 34(4): 471–78. DOI: 10.1080/09649069.2012.753733.

Leicester, M., and Cooke, P. (2002). Rights not restrictions for learning disabled adults: A response to Spiecker and Steutel. *Journal of Moral Education*, 31(2): 181–87. DOI: 10.1080/03057240220143287.

Mill, J. (1998). On liberty. In J. Gray (Ed.), *John Stuart Mill on liberty and other essays* (5–128). Oxford: Oxford University Press.

O'Callaghan, A. C., and Murphy, G. H. (2007). Sexual relationships in adults with intellectual disabilities: Understanding the law. *Journal of Intellectual Disability Research*, 51(3): 197–206. DOI: 10.1111/j.1365–2788.2006.00857.x.

Rojas, S., Haya, I., and Lazaro-Visa, S. (2014). *British Journal of Learning Disabilities*, 44: 56–62. DOI:10.1111/bld.12110.

Schormans, A. F., and Sobsey, D. (2017). Maltreatment of children with developmental disabilities. In M. L. Wehmeyer, I. Brown, M. Percey, K. A. Shogren, and W. L. A. Fung (Eds.), *A comprehensive guide to intellectual and developmental disabilities* (2nd ed., 509–26). Baltimore, MD: Paul H. Brookes Publishing Co.

Shogren, K. A., and Wehmeyer, M. L. (2017). Self-determination and goal attainment. In M. L. Wehmeyer and K. A. Shogren (Eds.), *Handbook of research-based practices for educating students with intellectual disability* (255–73). New York: Routledge.

Spiecker, B., and Steutel, J. (2002). Sex between people with "mental retardation": An ethical evaluation. *Journal of Moral Education*, 31(2): 155–69. DOI: 10.1080/03057240220143269.

Index

About the Authors

David F. Bateman, PhD (University of Kansas), is a professor at Shippensburg University in the Department of Educational Leadership and Special Education, where he teaches courses on special education law, assessment, and facilitating inclusion. Formerly, he was a due process hearing officer for over 580 Pennsylvania hearings. He uses his knowledge of litigation relating to special education to assist school districts in providing appropriate supports for students with disabilities. His latest area of research has been on the role of principals in special education. He has been a classroom teacher of students with learning disabilities, behavior disorders, intellectual disability, and hearing impairments, and a building administrator for summer programs. He has recently coauthored *A Principal's Guide to Special Education*, *A Teacher's Guide to Special Education*, and *Charting the Course: Special Education in Charter Schools*.

Thomas C. Gibbon, EdD, is chair and associate professor of the Department of Educational Leadership and Special Education at Shippensburg University. He earned an EdD in developmental education, curriculum instruction from Grambling State University, Louisiana, a MA in special education, and special education teaching certificates from McDaniel College, Maryland. He collaborates with two school districts to provide practice work sites at Shippensburg University for high school students with disabilities. He has published or presented on topics such as: the transition to adulthood and higher education for students with disabilities; sexual harassment and safety of SWD; sexual education for SWD; multicultural competence for preservice teachers; teaching children with chronic illness; inclusion; and family advocacy. Prior to his role in teaching preservice teachers, he worked with first-generation and underprepared college students, college students with disabilities, high school students with disabilities at a vocational technical school, and adults with disabilities going through the deinstitutionalization process.

Elizabeth A. Harkins Monaco, EdD, works as an assistant professor of special education at the University of Pittsburgh at Johnstown. Dr. Harkins received her BA from the University of Massachusetts at Amherst and obtained MA in special education at Lesley University in Cambridge, Massachusetts. She earned her PhD from American International College in Springfield, Massachusetts. Her experiences working in the field of special education include administration, teaching students with moderate to severe disabilities, and parent advocacy. Dr. Harkins's program of research is continuously evolving and emphasizes elements of holistic educational systems, specifically the importance of social justice and global citizenship alongside educational excellence for all students. She has also studied social and emotional development and diversity in special education, including the intersectionality of race and ethnicity with religion, gender, and sexual orientation for students with intellectual disabilities and autism spectrum disorders. Additionally, she has extensively studied and prepared presentations and manuscripts for emotional health, student-centered planning and self-determination, and sexuality education for students with intellectual disabilities and autism spectrum disorders. Dr. Harkins also works closely at the local, state, and national levels to improve the quality of life for persons with intellectual disabilities and autism spectrum disorders.

www.ingramcontent.com/pod-product-compliance
Lightning Source LLC
Chambersburg PA
CBHW030654270326
41929CB00007B/354